"This volume presents a broad and rich exploration of the many arenas in which psychoanalytic thinking can relieve suffering for patients and families. In it, internationally renowned analysts demonstrate how the psychoanalytic frame can be used to improve the lives of patients with a wide range of tenacious problems, from addiction to eating disorders to cancer, and in populations that range from the very young to those at the end of life. This book is a resource for those seeking to understand how the analyst's expertise can infuse medical care with much-needed humanism and wisdom."

Robert J. Waldinger, M.D. Professor of Psychiatry, Harvard Medical School. Director, Harvard Study of Adult Development

"Lest we take the fruitful convergence of psychoanalytic understanding and therapeutic relationship skills with day to day medical encounters that frame explorations in Balint groups for granted, in their chapter Lipsitt and Paulsen have provided the history of how this convergence developed from Freud to Ferenczi to Balint to today. Indeed, how psychotherapy and medicine have always been intertwined. In the process, they have reminded us, Balint group leaders and teachers of Balint group leaders, of the essential clinician patient relationship at the core of our current bio-psycho-social approach to patients and clients."

Laurel Milberg, PhD, past president and founding member of the American Balint Society

"The contribution to this collection by Randall Paulsen and Don Lipsitt is a major addition and rare synthesis of the 'enduring bridge between psychoanalysis and medicine'. The authors bring lifetimes of immersion in the study and practice of psychoanalysis and the Balint method to bear, as they review the pioneering work of Michael Balint and his eponymous seminars for practicing primary care physicians. Filled with detailed, readable, examples, the chapter is an opportunity to experience two experts as they think through the connections and ramifications of this 'bridge' between these cousins under the skin, medicine and psychoanalysis. The doctor-patient relationship is of course the bond they explicate, further instructing generations to come. You are in for a good and stimulating read."

C. Paul Scott, MD, DLFAPA; clinical professor of psychiatry, University of Pittsburgh School of Medicine; emeritus councilor and past-president, American Balint Society

"Finding meaning in physical illness is generally neglected by medical practitioners, but is often that which is sought by patients, consciously or unconsciously. When the illness affects children, the search for meaning becomes particularly painful. The present IPA volume is addressing these and other health struggles in various world settings. Case illustrations provide not only the 'feel' for lived experiences of both patients and health care professionals, but also serve as a model of psychoanalytic practice beyond the couch. This is an important contribution towards refreshing psychoanalytic thinking and thereby making it relevant to current complex times."
Astrid Berg, emerita professor, University of Cape Town, South Africa

"This engaging book contains descriptions of an interesting variety of clinical venues where application of psychoanalytic thought enhances medical care. It is a significant contribution to the emerging literature on this important subject. Areas covered include perinatology, pediatric inpatients, eating disorders, psycho-oncology, palliative care, addiction, and dermatology.

The principles described herein, applied to the increasingly technocratic practice of medicine, will help re-humanize it, providing necessary consideration to psychological factors that contribute to illness, psychological approaches that enhance management, and handling of adverse psychological reactions to illness and its treatment. This book will be of interest to medical students, doctors and nurses, as well as mental health professionals."
Paul Steinberg, MD, FRCPC, FIPA Clinical Professor, Department of Psychiatry, University of British Columbia

"Dr Harvey Schwartz and a diverse group of psychoanalytic thinkers bring us this comprehensive book to re-introduce George Engel, pioneer of psychosomatic medicine, Balint, Sandor Ferensczi and others and bring us back to present by focusing on the powerful interplay and intricate connection of psyche and soma both in health, illness and death. It takes the reader on a grand tour of major psychoanalytic viewpoints with a wide range of topics related to physical illnesses among children, adolescent and adults. They offer creative way of psychoanalytic understanding as well as technical intervention dealing with these group of patients. This timely book is well suited for psychoanalytic practitioners and medical professions to explore and become aware of potential transforming new paradigm."
Mali Mann, MD, FIPA; training and supervising psychoanalyst, USA

Applying Psychoanalysis in Medical Care

Applying Psychoanalysis in Medical Care describes the many ways that analysts interact with the medical world and make meaningful contributions to the care of a variety of patients.

Clinicians with a deep psychoanalytic understanding of our vulnerabilities, fears and hopes are well suited to participate in the care of our body. This book brings together contributions from caregivers who have dedicated themselves to deeply knowing their patients, from prenatal care, pediatrics, oncology and palliative care. The chapters are rich with moving clinical vignettes that demonstrate both the power and gracefulness of dynamic listening and insight.

This book will be valuable reading for psychoanalysts as well as practitioners and students in medicine, psychology, and the social work disciplines.

Harvey Schwartz, MD is a training and supervising psychoanalyst at the Psychoanalytic Center of Philadelphia and the Psychoanalytic Association of New York. He is a clinical professor of psychiatry and human behavior at the Sidney Kimmel Medical School, Thomas Jefferson University, Philadelphia, USA. He is the producer and interviewer for the IPA podcast, *Psychoanalysis On and Off the Couch.*

IPA in the Community

Series editor: Harvey Schwartz

Recent titles in the Series include:

Applying Psychoanalysis in Medical Care
Edited by Harvey Schwartz

Applying Psychoanalysis in Medical Care

Edited by
Harvey Schwartz

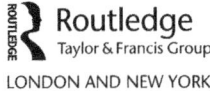
Routledge
Taylor & Francis Group

LONDON AND NEW YORK

First published 2022
by Routledge
2 Park Square, Milton Park, Abingdon, Oxon OX14 4RN

and by Routledge
605 Third Avenue, New York, NY 10158

Routledge is an imprint of the Taylor & Francis Group, an informa business

© 2022 selection and editorial matter, Harvey Schwartz; individual chapters, the contributors

The right of Harvey Schwartz to be identified as the author of the editorial material, and of the authors for their individual chapters, has been asserted in accordance with sections 77 and 78 of the Copyright, Designs and Patents Act 1988.

All rights reserved. No part of this book may be reprinted or reproduced or utilised in any form or by any electronic, mechanical, or other means, now known or hereafter invented, including photocopying and recording, or in any information storage or retrieval system, without permission in writing from the publishers.

Trademark notice: Product or corporate names may be trademarks or registered trademarks, and are used only for identification and explanation without intent to infringe.

British Library Cataloguing in Publication Data
A catalogue record for this book is available from the British Library

Library of Congress Cataloging-in-Publication Data
A catalog record has been requested for this book

ISBN: 978-0-367-76594-1 (hbk)
ISBN: 978-0-367-76593-4 (pbk)
ISBN: 978-1-003-16767-9 (ebk)

DOI: 10.4324/9781003167679

Typeset in Times New Roman
by Taylor & Francis Books

Dedicated to those psychoanalysts who enrich our world through working both on and off the couch

Contents

List of contributors	xi
Series Foreword	xv
IPA in Health Committee	xvi

Introduction   1
HARVEY SCHWARTZ

1 An incentive to use psychoanalytic psychosomatics in everyday medicine   6
JOACHIM KÜCHENHOFF

2 At a Crossroads: The Psychoanalytic Model and the Medical Model   24
KAREN PRONER AND VALENTINO AMMANNATI

3 On Becoming a Parent: When the Psychoanalyst Meets the Front-Line Professionals Involved in the Perinatal Period   36
MEROPI MICHALELI

4 Cruel Fate   51
JENNIFER DAVIDS

5 Day Hospital Intensive Care for Patients with Eating Disorders   71
HUMBERTO LORENZO PERSANO

6 Eating Disorders in Childhood and Adolescence: An Interdisciplinary Approach   91
MONICA ZAC, SANDRA NOVAS, LUZ MARÍA ZAPPA, JULIAN ONAINDIA, ALEJANDRA ARIOVICH AND ANDREA FRÄNKEL

7	Psychoanalysis and Psycho-oncology: How Each Specialty Enriches the Other NORMAN STRAKER	101
8	Psychodynamic Contributions to Palliative Care Patients and their Family Members LINDA EMANUEL	111
9	How a Lack of Human Connection May Lead to Dehumanization and Addiction JOSÉ ALBERTO ZUSMAN AND EDWARD J. KHANTZIAN	125
10	Psychoanalytic Approaches to the Skin Patient JORGE ULNIK	141
11	The Balint Group: The Arc of the Enduring Bridge between Psychoanalysis and Medicine RANDALL H. PAULSEN AND DON R. LIPSITT	161
	Index	190

Contributors

Valentino Ammannati, MD, graduated in medicine and surgery and specialized in pediatrics. He participated in a Balint group in his early career. He attended the first two years (the Observation Course) and two more years of the Development course of the Tavistock model child psychoanalytic training in Florence, Italy called Centro Studi Martha Harris. Presently, Dr. Ammannati, teaches in the pediatric training in the National Health Service of Tuscany.

Prof. Alejandra Ariovich, MD, is a pediatrician, specialized in adolescent medicine. She has been working as a member of the medical staff at the Adolescent Medical Service at the Hospital de Niños Ricardo Gutiérrez in Buenos Aires, mainly in the Inpatient Care Area. She has given several lectures and workshops on eating disorders. She belongs to the Adolescent Medicine Committee of the Argentine Society of Pediatrics, of which she is a full member.

Jennifer Davids, MSc (Clinical Psychology), is a child, adolescent and adult psychoanalyst who live and works in private practice in London. She has a long-standing interest in outreach work in the UK where she co-ordinated the British Psychoanalytical Society's group responding to the Grenfell fire, and in various projects in sub-Saharan Africa. She is the director of Africa Projects at the Children's Psychological Health Center, San Francisco. Jennifer trained in child and adolescent psychoanalysis at the Anna Freud Centre in London where she worked as a staff member, first as chief clinical psychologist and then on the teaching and analytic staff for 20 years. She also worked as a consultant child and adolescent psychotherapist in the National Health Service. Jennifer then trained in adult psychoanalysis at the British Psychoanalytical Society where she completed her fellowship. She is a supervising analyst for child and adolescent psychoanalysis. She is on the teaching faculty of the BPAS, has taught at the Tavistock, University College London, and the Maudsley Hospital. She teaches and presents internationally, and is currently working on a second book.

Linda Emanuel, MD, is an academic physician focused on palliative and end of life care. More than a decade ago she began training as a psychoanalyst alongside that. She is now professor emerita at Northwestern and in private practice as a psychoanalyst, still with a focus on people facing life-shortening illness or their family. She is a faculty member of the Chicago Psychoanalytic Institute and a member of the Boston Psychoanalytic Society & Institute.

Andrea Fränkel is a child and adolescent clinical psychologist. She is a staff member of the Mental Health Unit at Ricardo Gutiérrez Children's Hospital in Buenos Aires, working at the Inpatient Area. She is a professor at the University of Buenos Aires, School of Psychology.

Edward J. Khantzian, MD is professor of psychiatry (PT), Harvard Medical School, and a founding member of the Department of Psychiatry at the Cambridge Hospital. He has spent more than 40 years studying psychological factors associated with drug and alcohol abuse. Dr. Khantzian is a practicing psychiatrist and psychoanalyst, participant in numerous clinical research studies on substance abuse, and lecturer and writer on psychiatry, psychoanalysis and substance abuse problems.

Joachim Küchenhoff, MD, is a psychoanalyst (IPA, Swiss and German societies). He is a specialist in psychiatry, psychotherapy and psychosomatic medicine, professor emeritus of psychiatry and psychotherapy at the University of Basel, Switzerland, and visiting professor at IPU (International Psychoanalytic University) Berlin; he is president of the supervisory board at IPU and member of many other advisory boards. He is author and editor of many publications (www.praxis-kuechenhoff.ch).

Don R. Lipsitt is a professor of clinical psychiatry at Harvard Medical School, and chairman emeritus at Mount Auburn Hospital, Cambridge, Massachusetts. He has published over 100 articles, 26 book chapters, and four co-edited books. He has received numerous awards, including the Lifetime Achievement Award from the Association for Academic Psychiatry in 2001.

Meropi Michaleli, PhD, is a parent–infant and adult psychoanalyst. Her practice focuses on the psychoanalytic approach to pregnancy, infertility and the transgenerational transmission of presymbolic traumas. She led the implementation in Greece of the European Project "Naissance et Avenir" (Birth and Future), a training for health personnel involved in the perinatal and neonatal period who are faced with infants and families under high psychosocial risk. She is a member of the Hellenic Psychoanalytic Society and of the European Society for Child and Adolescent Psychoanalysis (SEPEA), founding member/former president of the Hellenic Society for Infant Mental Health (WAIMH Affiliate).

Sandra Novas, MD is a child and adolescent psychiatrist and a general psychiatrist. She is the head of the Mental Health Unit at Buenos Aires Hospital Ricardo Gutiérrez. She is a professor at the University of Buenos Aires, School of Medicine, Department of Psychiatry and Mental Health, where she is also the director of a specialization in child and adolescent psychiatry. She also works for the National Ministry of Health and has written and lectured widely on suicide attempts in adolescents.

Prof. Julian Onaindia, MD is a child and adolescent psychiatrist. He is a staff member of the Mental Health Unit at Ricardo Gutiérrez Children's Hospital in Buenos Aires, working at the Inpatient Area. He is a full member of the Argentinian Psychoanalytic Association (APA), IPA member and former section chief of the pediatric Emergency Department

Randall H. Paulsen, MD, is a psychiatrist, training and supervising psychoanalyst and past president of BPSI. He is an assistant professor of psychiatry at Harvard Medical School and currently supervises and consults at Brigham and Women's Hospital. His career has been focused on applied psychoanalysis, in directing inpatient and day hospitals at Tufts NEMC and Mt. Auburn Hospital (1981–1987), in developing primary care psychiatry as a component of Health Care Associates at BIDMC (1987–2000), and in facilitating a long-term Balint group for physicians. He was the mind-body consultant at the Osher Clinical Center at BWH where he also led mindfulness-based stress reduction courses (2002–2018). He views psychoanalysis as a subjective science in healthcare, human development and relationships (individual, group and institutional). He has a private practice of psychoanalysis in Lexington, Massachusetts.

Humberto Lorenzo Persano, MD, PhD, is training and supervising psychoanalyst at the Argentine Psychoanalytical Association (APA) and International Psychoanalytical Association (IPA), and general director of mental health services at the Ministry of Health in Buenos Aires. He is full professor psychology of nutrition and adjunct professor at the Department of Psychiatry and Mental Health, both at School of Medicine, University of Buenos Aires (UBA). He is a member of the IPA Health Committee and past co-chair for Latin America Committee on Psychoanalysis and the Mental Health Field (IPA).

Karen Proner, MS is a child and adult analyst. She is a member of IPTAR where she is on the faculty. She is a member of the IPA and APsaA. She has worked as a Consultant Child Psychotherapist in the National Health Service of Great Britain for many years. She runs a workshop in Rome and Florence, Italy on parent–infant work. She has been on the IPA committee for Psychoanalysis of Couples and Family. Presently, she is a member of the IPA in Health committee. She teaches and supervises in China, South Africa and Israel and has a private practice in New York

Harvey Schwartz, MD is a training and supervising psychoanalyst at the Psychoanalytic Center of Philadelphia and the Psychoanalytic Association of New York. He is a clinical professor of psychiatry and human behavior at the Sidney Kimmel Medical School, Thomas Jefferson University, Philadelphia. He is the producer and interviewer for the IPA Podcast, *Psychoanalysis On and Off the Couch*

Norman Straker MD is a clinical professor at Weill Cornell in the Department of Psychiatry, a consultant at Sloan Kettering Cancer Center and a faculty member of New York Psychoanalytic Institute. He is a distinguished life fellow of the American Psychiatric Association, and the author of two recent papers in the *Journal of Psychodynamic Psychiatry* and the editor of a book, *Facing Cancer and The Fear of Death: A Psychoanalytic Perspective on Treatment*.

Prof. Dr. Jorge Ulnik, MD, PhD, is a full member of the International Psychoanalytical Association, and training and supervising analyst at the Argentine Psychoanalytical Association. He is associate professor in pathophysiology and psychosomatic diseases at School of Psychology, Universidad de Buenos Aires, Argentina, and adjunct professor at Psychiatry and Mental Health Department School of Medicine, also at Universidad de Buenos Aires. He is president of the Euro-Latin American Psychosomatics School (EULAPS) and author of *Skin in Psychoanalysis* (Karnac, 2008).

Monica Zac, MD is a child and adolescent psychiatrist at Ricardo Gutiérrez Children's Hospital in Buenos Aires, where she coordinates the Inpatient Area of the Unit of Mental Health. Is a full member of APdeBA (Buenos Aires Psychoanalytic Association) and an IPA-certified child and adolescent psychoanalyst. She has been a member of IPA in Health since 2017 and she also acts as a liaison member between APDEBA and COWAP. She teaches and supervises individual and family psychotherapy.

Luz María Zappa, MD is a child and adolescent psychiatrist. She is a staff member of the Mental Health Unit at Ricardo Gutiérrez Children's Hospital in Buenos Aires, working at the Inpatient Area. She is an assistant professor at the University of Buenos Aires, School of Medicine, Department of Psychiatry and Mental Health.

José Alberto Zusman, MD, is chair of the IPA Subcommittee on Addiction, and post-doctor on addiction mentored by Edward Khantzian (Harvard). He is a full member and professor at the Psychoanalytic Society of Rio de Janeiro (SPRJ). He has a PhD in psychoanalysis, mentored by Eustachio Portella Nunus (Federal University of Rio de Janeiro). He is professor and supervisor of psychoanalysis at the Psychiatric Residency program at the Institute of Psychiatry, Federal University of Rio de Janeiro.

Series Foreword

I am pleased to welcome you to the IPA in the Community Book Series. These volumes will present the outreach work of the International Psychoanalytic Association as it integrates itself into many facets of our community life. We will learn how psychoanalysis, while born in the consulting room, also has application far beyond. Its core skills inform care provided to many individuals and in many venues from cancer units to refugee centers, from prenatal clinics to prisons. Through this book series we will get the opportunity to observe the deeply generous and skillful work of psychoanalysts who are making meaningful contact with individuals both on and off the couch.

Harvey Schwartz MD
Series Editor

IPA in Health Committee

Jennifer Davids, MSc
Admar Horn, MD
Joachim Kuchenhoff, MD
Humberto Persano, MD
Karen Proner MS
Yael Samuel, PhD
Norman Straker, MD
Monica Zac, MD

Introduction

Harvey Schwartz

Psychoanalysis is a deeply personal and nuanced method of treatment that offers the analysand the possibility of actualizing profound life changes. It enables an individual to have intimate contact with an other – a studied connection that awakens within themselves vibrant new potentials. These freedoms are born from insightfully experiencing the stasis of time that has unknowingly governed their lives. They come to recognize that they have been emotionally frozen in their pasts. Psychoanalysis liberates the present from this unrecognized past and in so doing enables new capacities for growth and maturation.

There are core psychoanalytic skills that are derived from this process that are applicable in venues and frames other than the analytic consulting room. We call this psychoanalysis "off the couch" – the use of a psychoanalytic attitude and basic interventions in service of offering individuals, and by extension communities, exposure to a new way of being heard. Being heard by a consistent and other-focused professional can itself open up new doors in one's life. For many, such hearing is a unique life experience. It not only facilitates a deeper capacity to listen to oneself. It also, through identification, enlarges one's ability to offer the same to others. It contributes to a chain of attentiveness and healing. Communities can be lifted by the buoyancy of insightful listening.

The International Psychoanalytic Association initiated a new program of outreach to the community under the presidential leadership of Dr. Virginia Ungar from Buenos Aires. The many newly established IPA in the Community committees have all brought their particular psychoanalytic vision to their respective areas of interest. This volume is a product of the IPA in Health committee. In it you will become acquainted with the work of experienced psychoanalysts who have applied their psychoanalytic skills in various medical settings.

In my following introduction to each chapter, I highlight how each psychoanalyst derives their interventions from a deep understanding of psychological development and the mind/body interface. More is involved though beyond cognitive understanding. Immersive listening to somatically

DOI: 10.4324/9781003167679-1

preoccupied individuals can elicit in the clinician a resonating attunement to their own body ruminations and tensions. A depth engagement both with ourselves and with those in our care asks a great deal from healers. What follows is the work of deeply attuned and talented psychoanalysts.

Küchenhoff, in the opening chapter "An Incentive to Use Psychoanalytic Psychosomatics in Everyday Medicine," offers a broad introductory embrace of psychoanalytic psychosomatics. He identifies the well-known temptations of dichotomous thinking – biology/mind – and provides in its place a three-dimensional healing encounter focused on the patient, not their symptoms, as the subject of the treatment. He describes the psychosomatic approach as "no longer a specialty that comes as the last resort after having tried everything else, but becomes an *attitude within medicine anew*" (emphasis added).

His chapter outlines the different effects of psychogenic struggles on the soma, the body as the enactor of unrecognized old object relationships, and the power of infantile trauma to remain as a haunting ghost in the cells of our physiology. The case presentations bring alive the challenges to and the growth that is possible when a transference relatedness is enabled. Somatic preoccupations can become transformed into interpersonal dramas. As the empirical data presented demonstrates, some affected patients emerge with a more vibrant capacity to live.

The creative tension between a dynamic and organic orientation towards those in our care is explicated in Proner and Ammannati's chapter, "At a Crossroads: The Psychoanalytic Model and the Medical Model." We get to know firsthand the struggles of a pediatrician who wishes to know and offer more to his patients beyond the prescription pad. This physician comes to recognize and tolerate a state of doubt. From there he becomes acquainted with its remedy either in the form of listening to his discomforts or placing blame on others. He honestly explores the attractions of each. He comes to appreciate, when working with children in pain, the power and usefulness of elaborating "the meaning of physical pain and transferring it on the mental plane." He explores for himself and his patients the space to observe, to think and to listen.

We experience the different form of this chapter, a report from a pediatrician, and learn as well of a different form of psychoanalytic education. The focus of the Centro Studi Martha Harris, the site of this training program in Florence, is the "emotional immersion in observation of a family and a newborn baby for two years." Such a setting facilitates the students developing "from not being able to imagine what another person might be thinking, to being able to form sensitive conjectures about a person's unconscious world." We too learn of a powerful model to introduce dynamic thinking and experiencing to our medical colleagues.

Michaleli, in her chapter, "On Becoming a Parent: When the Psychoanalyst Meets the Front-Line Professionals Involved in the Perinatal Period," describes her program in Athens where she establishes a novel benevolent presence into the lives of soon-to-be and new parents. She recognizes that a "yardstick for a civilized country is shaped by the measures and care practices applied for the protection of the health of pregnant women and newly born infants." Psychoanalysts appreciate that early caregiving is encoded in the body-to-body connection – the body is the medium of relatedness in the early days of life. The transgenerational transmission of mis attunement can be softened with the complimentary resilience of a responsive caretaker. The analytic facilitator invites parents to put their worries into words and thereby introduces a new relationship model into the rhythm of responsiveness. Parents firsthand recognition of this special presence attests to the power of these moments. A new father reflects:

> Their presence is what counts, and it is exactly by being present with you to attend the new little person that the conditions for accepting the baby for what she is are created... the memory of that experience is left within yourself as a beacon in the sky, and a man becomes a father by going back to it each and every tie the route is lost.

Davids, in her chapter, "Cruel Fate," describes her literal and internal journey as she becomes part of the complex workings of a hospital for children. She locates a geographic space for herself only to discover that her intrapsychic space will soon become filled to the brim with the projections of the suffering children, parents and staff. She encounters in others and describes for us in delicate and touching detail the all-too-common conviction that illness serves as warranted punishment. She and we learn that she herself must find respite and support from the unfairness of the sorrows. Cruel fate awaits many. Our appreciating the affective tolerance and skill of clinicians such as she is one of our all too temporary sources of solace in the face of those ever-present fates.

Persano, in his chapter, "Day Hospital Intensive Care for Patients with Eating Disorders," demonstrates how a disordered body-self representation serves as the final common pathway for an internal life characterized by weakened capacities for affect-regulation and mentalization and the tolerance of age-appropriate narcissistic vulnerabilities. A history of trauma often contributes to the experience of feeling like an inanimate object in the eyes of others which in turn becomes their own vision of themselves. A multi-disciplinary community-based treatment can function to challenge the malignant self-representations and can facilitate new internalizations and identifications. This can enable a more structured intra-psychic life and the maturation into an outpatient conflict-based therapy. Somatization can blossom into symbolization and with that an aggression imbued mirrored body image can soften into becoming a vessel capable of recognizing and embracing desire and love.

"No!" is the presenting organizing psychology of a 12-year-old anorexic boy described in Zac et al.'s chapter, "Eating Disorders in Childhood and Adolescence: An Interdisciplinary Approach." Like with many restricting patients, this "no" is recognized as not contributing to his development of an internalized subjectivity. It is a concrete "no" that lives outside the usual affective rhythms of adolescent relationships. It reflects his inability to meaningfully recognize inner desire as well as his mimicry of the interpersonal "no" of his non-attuned family environment. This "no" collapses the difference between inside and outside – he unconsciously provokes those around him as well as feels provoked by them. Hence, we learn of the necessity to therapeutically engage with both the individual and the family.

Even further, we learn of the long benevolent history of the hospital in which he is treated. Beginning in 1875 the Children's General Hospital Recardo Gutierrez in Buenos Aires has provided care for children. It provides a broad-based interdisciplinary team with which to engage all aspects of a child's life. This, in order to awaken the yearnings that hide in the absoluteness of this child's negativity. From this recognition of his authentic self he can then find words, conflicts and his own object directed "yes."

Straker, in his chapter, "Psychoanalysis and Psycho-oncology: How Each Specialty Enriches the Other," shares with us his early encounters with patients and families with cancer. His own analysis helped him struggle through his inclinations at that time to ally with the commonplace alienation and mechanization of these patients' medical treatment. Death anxiety, both the patient's and the physician's, had been denied and drained of informative meaning. He participated in the creation of the new sub-specialty of "psycho-oncology." He describes the foundations of "whole person medicine" which turns out to be the emotional forerunner of today's "personalized medical care." Character and defensive style are attended to, countertransference is recognized as ubiquitous and the positive transference is understood as bedrock to growth. Empathy comes to supplant denial, and omnipotence can soften to tolerating uncertainty. The clinical case demonstrates how this attentive care supports both a good life and a good death.

Emanuel shares her poignant perspectives on palliative care in her chapter, "Psychodynamic Contributions to Palliative Care Patients and their Family Members." She presents psychoanalytic concepts as they live in the moment in the time sensitive crucible of terminal illness. Her model of *existential maturity* serves as an umbrella under which she comes to view the adaptiveness of each person's manner of dying. Eschewing a judgement on maturity, she shares with us her appreciation of those internal factors that allow one to make meaning in the face of life's challenges. Such meanings, which are not linked to the chronological age of the dying, are born from a person's particular history of attachments, capacity for compassion and early caretaking. We get to meet two individuals whose deaths allow us a glimpse into what it means to be a psychoanalyst of the dying. It is psychoanalysis as it is always practiced – only more so.

Zusman and Khantzian invite us into the particular inner mind of those who suffer with addictions in their chapter, "How a Lack of Human Connection May Lead to Dehumanization and Addiction." They help us understand these patient's intolerance of dependency on others and how they suffer from a foundational experience of dehumanization. Their resultant facsimile of relatedness leads to their commonly attempted remedy of hyper-stimulation (i.e. drugs, food, sex, etc.). In a depth treatment the analyst will come to know of their patient's inner deadness by themselves being treated by them as an object of indifference. The analyst's capacity to recognize and tolerate this concrete counter-transference, often unaided by the buoyancy of symbolization, will determine the outcome of the treatment engagement. The authors provide a clinical master class on how one makes oneself therapeutically available to these struggling individuals.

Ulnik, in "Psychoanalytic Approaches to the Skin Patient," draws our attention to the multiple functions and meanings of our skin. It is the organ of interface with our physical environment and the carrier of our experience of being touched. It is the object of our gaze and the recipient of our self-abuse. We tattoo it, scratch it and exhibit it. This vehicle par excellence for somatic and psychic stimuli can best be therapeutically approached through joint dermatologic and psychologic interventions.

We learn of just such an approach in Dr. Ulnik's work. He and his dermatologist colleague both meet with the ailing patient and address the skin and also discover its psychic history. The goal is to quiet the inflammation and thereby set the stage for the emergence of words to represent affects. Thereby, an "allergic reaction to other people" can come to reveal the fear of and hope for the sought-after caress.

"Who has a case?" We learn in Paulsen and Lipsitt's chapter, "The Balint Group: The Arc of the Enduring Bridge Between Psychoanalysis and Medicine," that this is how a Balint group of physicians begin their meeting. This query sets in motion a group process of contained free associations. This will come to organize itself around a presenter who shares clinical details, discomforts and uncertainties on their care of a patient. The group members share their own reflections on the challenges of the case which stimulates new insights for the presenter on her relationship with the patient. The facilitator, addressing the group process and not the inner working of the presenter, helps synthesize the insights allowing the physician to transition from "feeling lost to feeling found."

The historical back story from which such a Balint group results is shown to begin in Budapest, in Michael Balint's home, with his general practitioner father. That and his intense later involvement with his analyst and then colleague Sandor Ferenczi led him to build upon Freud's emphasis on the "personality of the physician" in the delivery of medical care. He grew that notion to recognize that the *interaction* between patient and physician is at the core of the healing experience. The authors conclude that no less today in our era of genome specific treatments should the physician "lose sight of the necessity for all physicians to be comfortably skilled in addressing his or her patients' accompanying emotional response to virtually all disease."

Chapter 1

An incentive to use psychoanalytic psychosomatics in everyday medicine

Joachim Küchenhoff

Introduction

Ever so often, it has been heralded that by initiating biological therapies all psychological dimensions can be left out and forgotten. The detection of *Helicobacter* is a good example: as a consequence, virtually all clinical research on the psychodynamics of gastric ulcers which included methodologically impeccable empirical research (Weiner 1992) have been discarded. So searching the internet by the key words "gastric ulcer psychosomatics" will produce many results for ulcer, but in nearly all of them "psychosomatics" have been excluded. In line with that finding, an actual Wikipedia article on peptic ulcer states:

> While chronic life stress was once believed to be the main cause of ulcers, this is no longer the case. It is, however, still occasionally believed to play a role. This may be due to the well-documented effects of stress on gastric physiology, increasing the risk in those with other causes, such as *H. pylori* or NSAID use.
> (https://en.wikipedia.org/wiki/Peptic_ulcer_disease)

A more actual example would be gastric banding that indeed is effective in weight reduction but leaves the formerly adipose person alone with the effects of an extrinsically achieved change concerning the body image and the regulation of psychic homeostasis (Hsu et al. 1998).

In the domain of psychiatry, so called interventional methods are becoming predominant, like deep brain stimulation (Delaloye and Holtzheimer 2014) or ECT. They are applied as if they could supersede psychological approaches. It is quite normal for everyday psychopharmacology treatment not to monitor their subtler psychological implications below the threshold of established side-effects (e.g. the influence on concentration or on self-awareness and self-confidence).

What George Engel had in mind in the 1950s, to establish a psychosomatic-somatopsychic attitude in medicine, should not be forgotten but be re-introduced using modern psychoanalytic concepts:

DOI: 10.4324/9781003167679-2

Engel viewed the human organism as a psychobiological entity that is constantly open to influencing and being influenced by its environment and the people in it. He rejected the term 'psychosomatic disease' since it implies a special class of diseases of psychogenic aetiology, and asserted that the basic task of psychosomatic research is to identify psychosocial factors that alter individual susceptibility to any disease.
(Taylor 2002, p. 455; see also Engel 1967, 1974)

To consider individual susceptibility as an important factor entails to take into account the personality or the subjectivity of the patient. The German pioneer in psychosomatic medicine, Viktor von Weizsäcker, strongly advocated the "introduction of the subject" into medicine (cf. von Weizsäcker 1953, p. 50):

The true potential of psychosomatic medicine, Weizsäcker ventured, lay somewhere else entirely. The new medicine would have to stop considering organic disease/illness purely as an objective event – in the sense of an event that occurs in and as an object – and approach it instead in terms of questions that can only be asked of a subject, namely questions concerning motives, values and aims.
(Greco 2019, p. 111)

If we understand psychosomatic medicine as a medicine that in the sense of Engel or von Weizsäcker includes individual susceptibility or "the subject" in medical treatment, psychosomatic medicine no longer is a specialty that comes as the last resort after having tried everything else, but becomes an attitude within medicine anew.

The introduction of the subject into medicine does not exclude the body or the soma by any means. Soma and psyche cannot be isolated from each other, instead they are closely intertwined in any form of disease. Nevertheless, for heuristic purposes this psyche-soma interaction should be broken down into separable aspects:

First, the psycho-somatic effects: In psychoanalysis, psychic representations can often be traced back to interpersonal or intersubjective experiences; this holds true for many bodily expressions, as well. In clinical terms, the bodily symptom in many psychiatric disorders can often be interpreted and deciphered as a hidden form of addressing the significant other when the verbal interchange is blocked by various intrapsychic mechanisms. Psychoanalytic drive psychology, ego psychology, object relations theory and self psychology have contributed to an understanding of this infralinguistic "body talk".

Second, the somato-psychic effects that have to be considered in clinical practice. Take the clinical symptom of euphoria so often seen in disseminative encephalomyelitis patients; it is not necessarily a sign of a biological brain alteration but may be attributable to a defense operation in response to the severe and threatening disability. Take the severely anorectic patient as another example; the somatic status eventually leads to a (reversible) brain atrophy and, as a corollary, to many psychological disturbances, like a miscalculation of the body image.

In the beginning, psychosomatic medicine emerged from psychoanalytic sources or situated itself within the scope of psychoanalytic theory and practice. This linkage is no longer obvious. But still, it is worthwhile to have in mind the various models or concepts that have been forged in the heydays of psychoanalytic psychosomatics. These concepts are models that are valid and helpful in clinical practice in medicine. The search for "the" psychosomatic phenomenon or "the" psychosomatic patient has long been abandoned. This does not mean that the psychoanalytic concepts presented throughout the last hundred and more years have to be discarded. On the contrary: they are most valuable as models for the therapist to try to understand his or her psychosomatic patients. They do not allow to explain certain diseases specifically, but they *may* be useful in the encounter with the suffering individual. I have coined the term "constellative psychosomatics" (Küchenhoff 1994) to account for this epistemological turn in psychosomatics. Psychoanalytic concepts in psychosomatic medicine can be used as tools for the health professionals in the everyday encounter with a given patient.

Psycho-somatic effects

Models of Psychogenic Effects on the Body

Elsewhere I have outlined the most important models still valid in psychoanalytic psychosomatics on the influence of the psyche on bodily disease by using semiotic concepts, (i.e. the science of signs and signification) to classify the "body language" (Küchenhoff 2019). The overview presented here summarizes the models.

Conversion

Conversion signifies the transformation of mental energy into somatic innervation on the basis of a psychic conflict and by incorporation of these neuronal processes in expressive behavior – in such a way that the symptom has expressive content and can be deciphered in terms of body language. In the classical model of conversion hysteria, the drive conflict is oedipal; displacement onto the bodily level follows the pathways of the voluntary motor function and those of the senses; the outcome can be deciphered as a compromise-based enactment of the defense against oedipal wishes.

Sigmund Freud presented the first clinical and scientific account of a psychosomatic correlation in the model of conversion, which was, as we know, very successful in elucidating the causation of hysterical or hysteriform disorders. After considerable reflection, Freud remained totally within the province of psychology. This self-imposed limitation had consequences: the particular significance of psychoanalytic psychosomatics was initially to insist on establishing distinctions between the mental mechanisms contributing to the understanding of the psychosomatic transition, and this remains true to this day.

Affect Equivalents

Not every symptom is formed by conversion. Freud himself does not that all psychogenic body pathology is attributable to symbolization. (Freud and Breuer 1895, p. 179). The symptom then is not a symbol of a conflict, it does not represent it, but is merely an indication of it, assuming an indexical rather than a symbolic function. The index (forefinger or index finger) points to the designated object as does a physical forefinger to a physical object; it is a sign in the sense of an indication, a pointer; but there is no connection of content between the sign and what it designates. Freud calls this "conversion through simultaneity" (ibid., p. 178).

The realization of the indexical function of bodily symptoms is implicit in some important concepts of psychosomatic theory. One of these is the model of affect equivalents or affect correlates attributable to the psychoanalytic pioneer Otto Fenichel, a model applicable principally to somatoform disorders. We normally feel our emotional reactions as an integrated whole; emotions are experienced close to the body – that is, they are associated with bodily states. Now according to the model of affect equivalents, in a somatoform disorder disturbing mental events do not elicit integrated affective reactions. The functional affective reaction is preserved, while the mental ideas are repressed (Fenichel 1945). The sufferer may notice that "something is wrong"; the bodily symptoms can be deciphered as an indication of a psychic disturbance, but not as the condensed representation of a psychic conflict.

Alexithymia

In the early days of psychoanalytic psychosomatics, the conversion model was uncritically expanded. The symbolic interpretation of bodily processes increased beyond all limits, thus for a long time impairing the credibility of psychoanalytic psychosomatics. Freud himself countered this risk by contrasting the model of the actual neurosis with that of conversion. The former is not a psychoneurosis – that is to say, the psychic conflict is not processed and elaborated on the mental level – but arises in the immediate and present situation of a damming up of drives that cannot be relieved by a "specific or adequate action" (Freud and Breuer 1895, p. 108), so that the energy finds "abnormal employment" (ibid.) – namely, for the production of bodily symptoms such as vertigo or meaningless anxieties. Hence the paradigm of actual neurosis is characterized by the short-circuiting of the level of psychic representation and processing and the direct transformation of the mental conflict into bodily symptoms. This model of a somatic reaction due to an incapacity for psychic representation of experiences subsequently led to the model of alexithymia. The manifest inability of psychosomatic patients to describe their images of self and others in the clinical situation with appropriate affects and in differentiated form, their "disaffectation" (McDougall 1978) and norm-oriented, de-individualized narratives, suggest a need to investigate structural pathologies and ego restrictions in these patients. Nemiah and Sifneos (1970a, 1970b) termed the poverty of expression of affects "alexithymia," while Pierre Marty (1976) focused on exclusively technical and rational thinking (*pensée opératoire*), in which patients describe only external action situations, but not subjective attitudes and emotional impacts.

The alexithymia model suggests a deficit of representation in somatizing patients. The symptom assumes neither a symbolic nor an indexical function, but is meaningless and merely betokens a void in the context of the capacity for mental processing. However, the conclusion that a biological deficit underlies the alexithymic form of spoken communication is ultimately untenable. Alexithymic pathology can also be understood as a defensive process, albeit an archaic one. In this model the incapacity for representation is attributable to a destruction of representation, which is in turn always a psychic action and not a deficit.

The Body as a Locus for Enacting Relationships

Object-relations theory permits the investigation of unconscious ideas of the object; this is particularly fruitful where images of self and object are on the one hand modified and on the other transferred (e.g. projected). In severe personality disorders, such as those of the borderline type, ideas of self and object are split into dichotomized entities mostly in opposition to each other. In this way a threatening, confusing world of relationships is simplified and made readily comprehensible; polar black-and-white images replace complex differentiation of ideas of the self and graduated conceptions of other people. Since properties (e.g. good and bad ones) are thus no longer mixed together, good relationships that would otherwise be endangered by the dominance of destructive phantasies are preserved. The relevant point in psychosomatics is that the split-off images of self and others may be projected onto the body. A dialogue in the body then arises: a part of the body or the whole body is objectalized (treated as an object), and this part takes on properties of the object in the patient's phantasy. This projection onto the body is particularly significant in the dynamics of two pathologies – namely, hypochondria and self-harm.

Bodily Symptoms and Cohesion of the Self

Both hypochondria and self-harming behavior can also be seen as examples of the importance of the approach of self psychology to the understanding of bodily symptoms. The heightened concentration of attention on the body or bodily symptoms serves to enhance the experience of the body, and with it that of the self or ego, which is after all initially a bodily experience. In this way a reinforced sense of self can arise via the detour of increased cathexis of the subject's own body. This is relevant to all forms of psychopathology involving a threat to the sense of self. In patients suffering from diffusion of identity, as is typical of borderlines, the orientation (e.g. in hypochondria) to their body may constitute an attempt to regain cohesion of the self. The increased concentration of attention on the body intensifies the subject's experience of himself. In patients whose identity is under threat, a process of self-healing can be discerned in, for example, the formation of hypochondriacal symptoms: the looming fragmentation of the subject's self-image can be countered by hypercathexis of his body.

The Models' Practical Usefulness

The models presented above might be interesting for the specialized psychoanalyst as a starting point in therapy and for the scholars eager to understand better the mind-body-connectivity. I am deeply convinced that they can be useful for any physician or medical practitioner (MP), like a GP or a specialist for internal medicine, as well.

Acknowledging Psychogenetic Pathogenesis

The MP normally has been educated to think in pathophysiological and biochemical rather than psychological terms. Therefore, he or she tends to regard those phenomena that cannot be explained by biological causes as either factitious, simulated or stemming from unknown origins. Studying the models, he or she can get an idea of how the psychological mechanisms lead to bodily disturbances. By doing that, he or she might widen the etiological and pathogenetic concepts to encompass psychological motives and psychological causes.

Applying Psychogenesis as a Positive (Meaningful) Category

Psychosomatic diagnoses tend to be treated as residual categories that should be taken into account only after everything else has been excluded as a possible cause. The models allow to adopt an alternative attitude in showing that indeed there are positive criteria that lead to a psychosomatic diagnosis.

Contextualization of Symptomatology

Having in mind the psychoanalytically oriented models while talking to a patient, the MP has guidelines as to what he should include in his evaluation:

- Are there meaningful trigger situations prior to the onset of the symptomatology?
- Does the symptom have any expressive momentum?
- Are there additional signs and symptoms which may hint to an underlying personality disturbance, like artificial self harm, inadequate impulsivity and others?
- What about the capacity of the patient to be introspective and to verbalize personal feelings?
- Does the symptomatology convey a considerable secondary gain?

Fostering the Doctor–Patient Relationship

Somatoform disorders are widespread and arguably the diagnostic group with the highest incidence rate in general practice. These patients may ask for repetition of diagnostic interventions, as is typical for patients with hypochondriasis, and they will be disappointed ever so often. The doctor in his or her turn will be annoyed as he or she feels manipulated or devaluated by the patient. Then the therapeutic relationship between the MP and the patient is in danger. If the patient instead feels addressed as a person with individual and subjective experiences, thoughts and feelings, he or she will develop or regain trust in the MP as a confidant person.

Case Example

The models differentiated in the section above should not be conceptualized as alternatives so that only one would be applicable to any one patient. As models they do not represent the "real" disease processes but are tools for understanding the psychodynamics of a given disease. So in the course of a psychotherapy, different models might be adequate. This will be shown in the case vignette now. At the same time, it serves as an illustration of how the models can be applied in therapeutic practice.

I give a brief account of my first interview with Mrs. A. She is extremely thin (BMI of under 17). She is self-controlled and at the same time reflective in her descriptions, emotionally reserved; only at the end, when we talk about the lost professional aspirations, tears roll down her cheeks. With all her friendliness in contact, it is not easy to feel what she actually wants to achieve for herself.

Mrs. A has been through a lot of therapy. Nevertheless, she is convinced to need more, her main motivation being the persisting difficulty in self-care expressing itself in her eating habits. She then describes an eating behavior as is typical for anorexia nervosa. The anorexia developed after a bout of depression at the age of 20, she lost appetite during depression and only afterwards adopted an anorexic illness behavior. It has been a great concern for her to not gain a foothold professionally. Another major problem are the recurring states of tension which she cannot cope with herself so she has felt forced to drink alcohol or take psychopharmaceutic drugs.

Mrs. A went to a secondary grammar school, then to university and finally completed her specialist training. The aforementioned depressive and anorexic crisis stopped her professional career. She now has a sheltered job as a shop assistant. She has been living in a therapeutic residential community where she is on her own, but shares meals with her flatmates three evenings a week.

Her father was a civil engineer; he was in charge of an own plant. He always worked a lot, being an introverted person. The factory finally went bankrupt. That was a hard blow for him from which his self-esteem never recovered. Mrs. A. had great difficulties with her mother, she was used (and abused) by her as the main contact person, as father was hardly ever available. Mother demanded that everything should be kept inside the family and never be confided to persons outside. Mother had a serious alcohol problem, but never underwent therapy. She was very rigid and could only look after herself. Mrs. A maintains that she learned early on to look after herself and never showed anyone how she really felt. She recalls a restless childhood interrupted ever so often by relocations in the country or abroad due to father's professional obligations or aspirations.

She is the eldest of the children, she has always been particularly fond of her younger sister, they had a close relationship, but the sister finally withdrew from her because of the patient's longstanding eating disorder. Contrary to Mrs. A, all siblings are married meanwhile and have children on their own.

Mrs. A is highly ambivalent about her mother. From an early age she has been annoyed by her mother's permanent complaining about her own ailments without having an ear for the daughter's worries. At the same time, the mother remained helpless, dependent on the help of others, and mainly of her eldest daughter, due to an alcohol addiction. Separating from the family in adolescence and later on always meant for Mrs. A abandoning her mother and in a way let her die. The three siblings who followed quickly had to be supported during childhood. Instead of being cared for herself, she looked after the siblings instead of the mother, who often was drunk and unavailable. A father, who would triangulate the relationships as an alternative object and relieve the dependence on the mother, was not at hand. The real father remained entangled in his professional conflicts.

In therapy, I feel committed to Mrs. A. But the dilemma of care and self-sufficiency is quickly repeated in our therapeutic relationship. I feel the urge to help Mrs. A, she seems to rely on my support, but without in any way distancing herself from the sometimes delusionally fixated self-command to continue losing weight. If her low weight forces me to admit her to a hospital, I am no longer the therapist who protects her and cares for her, but the object that drops her, that knows no consideration.

Mrs. A obviously suffers from a serious personal problem, which is connected to the conflict between a desire for care on one side and the wish for autarky on the other, according to the diagnostical OPD system (Operationalized Psychodynamic Diagnostics; OPD Task Force 2001). The anorectic symptomatology, the anorectic handling of food has a strong expressive and symbolic character (cf. conversion). In dealing with the food the care-autarky-conflict is always represented and re-enacted anew. On the one hand, the completely starved body shows the neediness and expresses an appeal that cannot be formulated in words: "Take care of me!" At the same time, however, autarky or self-sufficiency predominates: Mrs. A rejects any support that could lead to a normalization of her weight.

In the course of therapy, the psychodynamic quality of the anorectic behavior changes and for a while cannot be interpreted as a symbolic representation of an intrapsychic conflict. As the therapy moves on, the therapeutic relationship intensifies, Mrs. A now feels more and more dependent on me, symbiotic and merging phantasies become prominent and provoke anxieties as to lose the boundaries between herself and me as the transferential object. To shelter herself from the dissolution of the self, she becomes alexithymic meaning that she feels herself exhausted, without phantasy, void, without words, she retreats from the therapeutic dialogue into a sort of psychic numbing where she does not have to feel anything (cf. alexithymia). The anorectic behavior then supports the foreclosure, the radical exclusion of psychic representation; the feeling of being hungry all the time becomes dominant and bans all other forms of psychic representation. It is only by repeatedly interpreting the regressive transferences that this merger state of structural regression can be overcome. Working through the level of fusionary object relations in the transference turned out to be the pivotal point in therapy helping Mrs. A to understand and overcome the emotional entanglement with her mother which was reactivated in all closer and personal relationships.

Conclusion: Psychoanalytic models in psychosomatic medicine offer tools to understand the dynamics of body – related psychic symptoms in a broad variety of psychiatric disorders. They can be helpful to see in how far the body "speaks" for the person who is incapable to express wishes, emotions and thoughts by verbal language. As the case report shows, the models do not only differentiate between diagnostic groups but are suited to monitor different phases during therapy with the same patient.

Somato-psychic Effects: Ways of Coping with a Disease from a Psychoanalytic Point of View

Acute and severe somatic illnesses inflict severe psychological stress for the patient. The disturbance of bodily well-being has a serious impact on the narcissistic investment of the body. Thus a vital dimension of self-coherence is called into question. Being confronted with the diagnosis of a chronic disease implies that future life perspectives have become insecure, since the patient must live with the danger of possible relapse or even death. He or she faces unusual dependencies on medical professionals and medical treatment. Therefore confrontation with an acute or chronic illness constitutes a challenge to the personality and its adaptive resources. This will be shown by case examples first and by a summary of a qualitative empirical research study.

Case Studies

Somatic Disease as a Trauma: Psychic Decompensation Due to an Acute Illness

I have known Mrs. B, a very intelligent and adroit woman in her late sixties, for a couple of years now. She started therapy with me because she became severely depressive and even had to be treated in a psychiatric hospital before. Prior to the depressive crisis, a project of high personal importance had failed: together with her partner, she had invested a lot of money in the acquisition of a stately mansion which was to be used professionally but also kindled her hopes to finally find a home for her own. Not to feel at home anywhere turned out to be her basic attitude to life.

Mrs. B was given away for adoption as a very small baby. Her adoptive parents were well to do but did not at all get along with each other; so the adoptive father soon had extramarital sexual relationships, and the adoptive mother slowly but irreversibly became addicted to alcohol. Mrs. B was left to herself or the house servants during childhood.

Due to her vivid temperament and her intellectual abilities she finished school and a university course. After her adoptive parents died shortly after another when she was in her twenties she was confronted with a rich inheritance, but without any personal support. She married soon and had a first child, but the marriage did not last long. A second marriage turned out to be much more durable and persists till today. With her second husband she had another child.

In 2020, when the COVID-19 infection was spreading, she caught the virus and fell severely ill. She could no longer breathe properly and was in panic about suffocation. She refused to enter an ICU, isolated herself and had her medical treatment at home, in an isolated room within her house. Nevertheless, she consequently stuck to the quarantine rules. I could only maintain the therapeutic talks via online video conferences.

Within days of the seclusion, Mrs. B became more and more lightheaded, logorrheic, agitated, and in the end showed all signs of a manic episode. She denied all my suggestions to allow an anti-manic psychopharmacological regime and strongly accused me to hinder her from finally being able to live a consequent and fruitful and vital life. She felt to be complete and self-sufficient for the first time in her life. She announced to end the therapeutic relationship with me, parallel to severing the contact to her husband and her daughter living in the same or the adjacent villa. In the end, she always maintained the video talks even though sometimes she went online only up to 15 to 20 minutes late.

My countertransference feelings were strong and difficult to endure. At times I was in doubt about the legal consequences: should I not transfer her to a psychiatric hospital even against her will because she was endangered somatically and socially? I monitored her psychopathological status again and again but always decided against any unwanted interference. Other times I felt insulted and got very angry and unwilling to accept the denigrations and attacks, so I tended to stop the seemingly futile talks. In the end I persevered, and both Mrs. B and I have now been able to resume therapy in the ordinary setting enabling us to reflect on what happened during the infection period.

Why did Mrs. B become psychotic? Meanwhile she has been able to describe in detail how the restrictions in breathing caused severe anxieties to die. The first trauma interfering with the hitherto functional level of structural integration of the personality was the danger of an imminent death. There was a second trauma interfering with the first, the revival of a very early trauma, the trauma of being abandoned and entirely on her own. The manic state can best be understood as a reversal or a reaction formation: with the help of the manic feelings, she could feel completely independent, superior to others because she felt she no longer needed anyone. Instead, she was able to frighten others, including me, causing them to depend on her.

Conclusion: This case vignette shows how deeply an acute and threatening illness might destabilize the ego strength and cohesion of the personality. On the other hand, it allows to understand the response, pathological though it may appear, as a meaningful counter to the traumatic situation.

Chronic Disabling Illness, Illness Behavior and the Issue of the So-called Non-compliance

Mr. C was referred to me a year ago by a neurological outpatient clinic. There, the medical personnel had been infuriated and angry because Mr. C would not accept the appropriate treatment of his progressive encephalomyelitis disseminata (MS), neither with corticosteroids nor with modern biologicals.

Mr. C is 60 years old. He needs crutches to be able to walk a short distance as the MS has affected the legs predominantly whereas his arms are much less afflicted. In our second talk, he lifts himself up from the chair in the consultation room too fast and tumbles to the floor. He won't be helped up and insists on standing up himself. He speaks in a loud voice; far from being impressed by the chronic illness or the stage of disability he is in a fighting spirit. He devalues his neurologists who dare to try to enforce a treatment that he is not willing to accept. He claims he has found an alternative way by following the Coimbra protocol (www.coimbraprotocol.com) and by exercising yoga. Similar to so many other patients suffering from MS, he expects psychoanalytic psychotherapy to halt the disease progression.

Mr. C is married to a somewhat younger woman whom he encountered on a trip in another continent. Whereas he hardly can help himself and is in need of her support, he constantly criticizes her and exposes a condescending attitude towards her, this behavior leading to many fights between the partners. He obviously feels superior to her, notwithstanding his disability.

Somehow he has come to accept me as a therapist. This may be partially due to the fact that I do not feel inclined to follow the neurologists' demand to re-establish compliance. On the one side, I am impressed by his stubbornness; on the other side I consider his illness behavior as irresponsible towards himself and his wife. I am curious to know why he denies the help he so urgently needs and why he relies on a therapy without proven effectiveness.

Soon we talk about his relationship to his mother who is only 20 years older. Up to the present day, she is not capable to listen. She has overwhelmed her son all the time with her own health-related or personal issues. She never has let him follow his own way but always has known beforehand what is helpful or detrimental for him. Though he is loud and self-assertive in communication with others, he cannot stop her or make himself visible or hearable in front of her.

For me, it is difficult to say anything meaningful because Mr. C fills the therapeutic sessions with never ending stories on his daily businesses. I feel pushed back and held at a distance. It becomes evident in the long run that Mr. C is identified with his mother inducing in my (concordant) countertransference the feelings he ever so often has had: not being able to make oneself seen and taken into consideration. After having worked through this important pattern in the object relationship the permanent quarrels in the marital relationship subside; they had been governed by the same pattern of role reversal and projective identification.

Only then are we able to understand together that it is impossible for him to follow the neurological prescriptions. He cannot see in them a chance for help; he hears – as it were – his mother's unrelenting monologues and must by any means maintain his personality by declining the offered treatment, a personality that is endangered so much by the loss of motor neuron control and other disabilities. As a consequence, Mr. C now is willing to examine the chances implicated in the actual neurological treatment schemes.

Conclusion: What has a psychoanalytic approach to offer in coping with a chronic disease according to this case example? Analyzing the habitual and sometimes dysfunctional object relations and the personality traits of the person who has to face a chronic illness helps to elucidate and understand the disease process and the predominant coping forms. Eventually it helps to improve the doctor – patient – relationship which is burdened by a severe disagreement about what is indicated. It obviously does not improve the compliance as the patient will not comply more readily and will not follow unequivocally the medical advice, but it may help to foster a mutually respectful and trustful relationship.

Empirical Research

Following the case study approach, the somato-psychic dimension is now elaborated on a wider scale by a short description and summary of a part of an empirical research project that I had the chance to perform together with a powerful research team. The complex project lasted more than 7 years and was completed almost 20 years ago. Some of the data are still valid and worth being discussed. Therefore I enclose the part that is pertinent to the scope of this chapter.

The Heidelberg Research Project on Crohn's Disease

The Heidelberg Research Project on Crohn's Disease (Küchenhoff 1993a, 1993b) was a longitudinal study that analyzed the interrelation of personality, defense and coping in the course of Crohn's disease. Crohn's disease is a severe and chronic relapsing illness mainly of the gastrointestinal tract; the patients suffer from abdominal pain, bloody diarrhea, fistula formation and severe impairment of general health. Various extraintestinal manifestations may complicate the picture.

The project design ran as follows. Acute illness, the criterium for being included in the sample, was defined as a disease activity of more than 150 points in the Crohn's Disease Activity Index (CDAI). The patients were seen a second time, when the disease process had reached remission; remission was defined as a disease activity of less than 100 points in the CDAI; corticosteroid medication had to be reduced to less than 10 mg prednisone and no immunosuppressive therapy was allowed. Those patients who did not recover were seen 12 months after the first assessment. They were revisited a third time three years after the first interview. In the intervals, contact with the patients was maintained by means of a questionnaire concerning their somatic state; these were sent on a monthly basis until remission and after that every four months. These questionnaires and the data drawn from the medical charts in phase 1 and from a final medical examination in phase 3 were the information we had on the patients' somatic state. In each phase, a psychological testing was performed; two questionnaires were psychological and psychodynamic personality inventories, others were used to assess the patients' defense style, their coping and their happiness with life.

Many subjective experiences cannot be read from questionnaires such as the emotional response to the illness, biographic facts and the actual social and psychological adaptation to life; we therefore did not restrict ourselves to the questionnaires and carried out psychodynamic interviews with the patients in phase 1 and 2; these interviews were recorded and were the basis for a complex rating of defense mechanisms and for content analyses in 50 patients.

It is fortunate that qualitative research today has attained a high methodological standard thus allowing its acceptance within the scientific community. It allows a livelier picture of how the patients cope with the disease. We found five different types of subjective answers to the disease which served as an illustration for the statistical analyses. Overtly depressive or dysthymic patients tended to regard *the illness as a reinforcement of their negative approach to life*. A depressive personality structure and the burden of the acute or chronic ailment can initiate a vicious circle ending in what psychoanalysts may call an ego regression or what could be described as an assimilation to the illness state. Anxieties may generalize in the course of the disease; realistic fear may be converted into panic attacks. Bodily self-awareness may disintegrate; the patients feel subjected to uncontrollable bodily processes. Demands and hopes in everyday life and for the future are lowered and reduced. The patient's life is devoted to self-pity and a reproachful attitude towards others.

In patients that regard achievement and success as vital for their self-esteem the disease may interfere very much with the high personal aspirations. Some patients decide to let themselves not be disturbed by the disease at all. I have coined the label "Business as usual: the non-reactive type" to characterize a risky type of adaptation that could be found mostly in men; these outwardly energetic patients do not adapt at all to the disease, they present themselves as if they could live their lives in the customary way even if they are dangerously ill. Denial has become excessive here; no psychic changes occur parallel to the changes from the acute illness and its stress to recovery. Because denial of the disease is strong throughout, the illness cannot initiate a psychological development or even growth; on the contrary, the over-compensating attitude will be enhanced by the disease process.

The types described so far are characterized by little flexibility in coping with the disease process. In others much more variability can be found. For one adaptive type the term "pseudo-autonomous development" was coined. Patients showing this kind of adaptation had been confronted with demands for separation and individuation before getting ill. Some patients felt tormented by the already described loyalty conflicts, mainly between parents and sexual partner. They fell ill while this in-between constellation was yet unsolved; they took the illness serious, even as a challenge to change their hitherto lifestyle. But they did not proceed to become more autonomous; they solved the interpersonal conflict by giving up their friendship and were happy to regain a harmonious relationship with their parents.

By now, it seems that negative courses of coping with Crohn's disease prevailed. We saw others where the disease was taken seriously without impeding or worsening personal development, on the contrary it was even enhanced. I was especially impressed by those patients who took the disease as a stimulus to give up a very one-sided lifestyle characterized by overwork, emotional rigidity and a denial of personal bounds, in order to accept the more sensitive and demanding parts of their own personality. These patients could, in other words, integrate experiences formerly denied; I have named this type of adaptation "regression in the name of the ego".

The fifth type of adaptation demonstrated the most astonishing psychic development. I have used the term "integrative course" for this type. For these patients, the acute disease had been traumatic in the sense of the word; the ego had been overwhelmed and had been incapable of coping with the various moments of distress and threats. Fear of dying or psychic disintegration prevailed. These patients could not protect themselves by denial; it becomes evident here that – as we have seen in reviewing the results of discriminant analysis – a certain degree of denial in an acute crisis is necessary and sound. In the course of the disease process, these patients were able to mourn, to work through their fears and threats and acknowledge the changed life perspective without being paralyzed or knocked down. A new balance was achieved that was regarded by the patients themselves as a change for the better even when compared to the psychological state before illness. Here is a short case report.

Mrs. D was in despair when she fell acutely ill. She spoke of a "complete life panic":

> To go to the doctor and to admit I have to take the disease serious that I cannot understand and will not understand. Life has become a catastrophe: to raise one's head that can't stop thinking and questioning everything. Most of my perspectives have been destroyed.

At that time the patient was desperate (even suicidal), reproachful and self-destructive.

During the time of recovery she found a different way of talking about herself; in remission she was more thoughtful and respectful, ready to look after herself, but also more ready to see and acknowledge others. While in acute illness she experienced her body as a source of constant threat ("I know, if I can overcome Crohn's disease I'll get cancer"), in remission, she could handle herself with care for the first time in her life. "What I take Crohn's disease for, is to take care and do something. In the hospital, I practiced what was good for me: taking a bath, taking drugs regularly, which I had detested before. It has become better and I have a feeling of well-being now."

In her biography, this patient had been confronted with serious handicaps early on. From the start, she had to share everything, especially her parents' love, with a twin brother; an elder sister had been born with a severe genetic malformation and demanded most of her parents' time. Both parents were teachers and devoted most of their pedagogic skills to the handicapped child. A small brother was born when the patient was five years; he soon became everyone's "pet", the much-preferred youngest child. Delegating her devotion to her grandmother, the patient tried to overcome strong feelings of jealousy. But the grandmother died when she was fourteen; she decompensated and became an alcoholic until the outbreak of Crohn's disease. She tried to find friends and began a symbiotic relationship to a woman who she needed as sexual partner, mother and grandmother and even more; of course this friend could not fulfil all the claims, she separated from the patient who fell ill soon afterwards.

Only by understanding this biography can one imagine why separation could be so traumatic. The illness itself reinforces feelings of loneliness, being abandoned and feeling dependent. What is impressing nevertheless is the fact that the breakdown of psychic integration at the stage of acute illness can be reversed during the course of the illness. The patient can experience self-pity and self-care, the illness serves as a means to take care of herself. In psychoanalytic terms, the patient becomes able to identify herself with her caring and mothering grandmother and therefore can take on mothering functions for herself. The capacity for concern that was projected onto others before the onset of the disease could now be internalized.

Concluding Remarks

Coming close to the end of this chapter, I want to summarize its main propositions. As the title announces, it wants to stimulate the use of psychoanalytic psychosomatics in everyday medicine. This can be done using two main approaches, a psychosomatic and a somatopsychic pathway. It may be clearer to insert a dash into the composite terms; a psycho-somatic perspective focuses on the impact of psychological factors on bodily wellbeing, whereas the complementary perspective, the somato-psychic one, studies the effects that a change in the somatic status has on the psyche. Both aspects are intertwined with each other in a network of intercorrelations between mind and body. Obviously, up to now there is no mind without a body and no body without a mind. They are one entity, and it is only for analytic purposes that they are taken as separate entities. Thus, specific effects can be described in isolation from other influences. But in the end, they have to be regarded in their complex interactions.

Sometimes, the psycho-somatic and the somato-psychic dimensions are mixed up. For instance, the distortions of the body image in anorexia nervosa were seen for a long time as signs of the underlying identity diffusion reaching the body; meanwhile, it is acknowledged as a somato-psychic consequence that improves automatically as soon as the weight is restored to normal.

In the early twentieth century, psychosomatic medicine was more or less identical with psychoanalytic psychosomatics. As psychoanalysis has lost its ubiquitous influence this is no longer the case. So, psychoanalysis has to prove its values in competition with other, mainly cognitive-behavioral concepts. Especially the somato-psychic perspective has been more or less successfully taken over by cognitive-behavioral psychology (i.e. the coping approach). Still, psychoanalytic concepts are extremely useful in linking the forms of coping with or defense against acute or chronic illnesses to life-long experiences that mold the individual perception of the illness.

As to the psycho-somatic perspective, psychoanalysis has been criticized and oftentimes superseded not by psychological alternatives, but by biological etiologies and pathophysiological pathways. A lot of empirical research data has been neglected showing and proving the impact the psyche might have on the body. To be sure, psychoanalytic reasoning tended to be one-sided itself omitting the complexity of the biological side. But this does not justify a negligence the other way round. At any rate, psychoanalysis allows to introduce the subject into medicine in its undiminished complexity including both conscious and unconscious experiences, attitudes and ways of thinking.

Is psychoanalysis too demanding and complex for being useful in everyday medicine? The models introduced in the first part of this chapter are not self-descriptive, and they predispose a certain familiarity with psychoanalytic concepts. But that does not speak against the models' practicability. Otherwise, other treatment principles, for instance pharmacology, would encounter the same critique. So a certain amount of expertise is mandatory. But on the other hand, even the MP not having been trained in psychoanalytic or psychodynamic reasoning can profit from the models by having in mind the dimensions of subjectivity involved in the diagnostic and therapeutic work.

I wish to end the chapter with a quote from the Greek philosopher Aristotle who strongly opposed dualistic thinking and regarded the soul as the form of the body. He states:

> It is not necessary to ask whether soul and body are one, just as it is not necessary to ask whether the wax and its shape are one, nor generally whether the matter of each thing and that of which it is the matter are one. For even if one and being are spoken of in several ways, what is properly so spoken of is the actuality.
> (*De Anima* ii 1, 412b6–9, trans. Hicks 1907)

The quote underlines that the psyche and the body belong to each other in a complex way and that the practical need to discriminate the parts, like the psycho-somatic and the somato-psychic perspective, should not mislead us to adopt a narrow dualistic approach.

References

Delaloye, S. and Holtzheimer, P. (2014) Deep Brain Stimulation in the Treatment of Depression. *Dialogues in Clinical Neuroscience* 16(1): 83–91.

Engel, G. L. (1967) The Concept of Psychosomatic Disorder. *Journal of Psychosomatic Research* 11: 3–9.

Engel, G. L. (1974) Memorial Lecture: The Psychosomatic Approach to Individual Susceptibility to Disease. *Gastroenterology* 67: 1085–1093.

Fenichel, O. (1945) *The Psychoanalytic Theory of Neurosis*, 3 vols. New York: Norton.

Freud, S. and Breuer, J. (1895) *Studies on Hysteria*. Standard Edition of the Complete Works of S. Freud, Vol. 2. Richmond: Hogarth Press.

Greco, M. (2019) On illness and Value: Biopolitics, Psychosomatics, Participating Bodies. *Medical Humanities* 45: 107–115.

Hicks, R. D. (trans.) (1907) *Aristotle: De Anima*. Cambridge: Cambridge University Press.

Hsu, L., *et al.* (1998) Nonsurgical Factors That Influence the Outcome of Bariatric Surgery: A Review. *Psychosomatic Medicine* 60(3): 338–346.

Küchenhoff, J. (1993a) *Psychosomatik des M. Crohn: Zur Wechselwirkung seelischer und körperlicher Faktoren im Krankheitsverlauf* [*Psychosomatics of Crohn's Disease: The Interaction of Psychological and Somatic Factors during the Course of the Disease*]. Stuttgart: Enke.

Küchenhoff, J. (1993b) Defense Mechanisms and Defense Organizations: Their Role in Adaptation to the Acute Stage of Crohn's Disease. In U. Hentschel, G. Smith, W. Ehlers and J. Draguns (Eds.), *The Concept of Defense Mechanisms in Contemporary Psychology* (pp.412–424). Berlin: Springer.

Küchenhoff, J. (1994) Spezifitätsmodelle in der psychosomatischen Medizin – Rückblick auf eine alte Kontroverse [Models of Specificity in Psychosomatic Medicine – Looking Back to a Longlasting Controversy]. *Zeitschr f Psychosom Med und Psychoanal* 40: 236–248.

Küchenhoff, J. (2019) Intercorporeity and Body Language: The Semiotics of Mental Suffering Expressed through the body. *IJPA* 100(4): 769–791.

Marty, P. (1976) *Les mouvements individuels de vie et de mort* [*Individual Life and Death Movements*]. Paris: Payot.

McDougall, J. (1978) *Plea for a Measure of Abnormality*. New York: International Universities Press.

Nemiah, J. C. and Sifneos, P. E. (1970a) Affect and Phantasy in Patients with Psychosomatic Disorders. *Modern Trends in Psychosomatic Medicine* 2: 26–34.

Nemiah, J. C. and Sifneos, P. E. (1970b) Psychosomatic Illness: A Problem in Communication. *Psychotherapy and Psychosomatics* 18: 154–160.

OPD Task Force (2001) *Operationalized Psychodynamic Diagnostics: Foundations and Manual*. Seattle, WA: Hogrefe.

Taylor, G. (2002) Mind–Body–Environment: George Engel's Psychoanalytic Approach to Psychosomatic Medicine. *Australian and New Zealand Journal of Psychiatry* 36: 449–457.

von Weizsäcker, V. (1953) *Der Gestaltkreis*. Frankfurt: Suhrkamp.

Weiner, H. (1992) *Perturbing the Organism: The Biology of Stressful Events*. Chicago, IL: University of Chicago Press.

Chapter 2

At a Crossroads

The Psychoanalytic Model and the Medical Model

Karen Proner and Valentino Ammannati

Introduction (by Karen Proner)

I have been very fortunate to have taught in Florence, Italy, for forty years in a psychoanalytic psychotherapy training center for child and adolescent therapists. It is based on the Tavistock model for the child psychotherapy training in London. The head of the original center, Esther Bick, and John Bowlby, established the center in 1948 to train non-medical people to fill the new British National Health Service Child Guidance Clinics with child psychanalytic psychotherapists to see children and families. Martha Harris succeeded Mrs. Bick and continued to develop this training center into a premier center for child psychotherapists with the same rigorous training requirements of the child analytic training centers in the psychoanalytic institutes. For this reason, its reputation grew throughout Europe. Martha Harris and her husband Donald Meltzer began traveling to Italy teaching and supervising and by the 1980s they had established a training in different cities of Italy, starting with Florence. Now there are Tavistock model child analytic training centers all over Italy. The one in which I have been faculty is in Florence Italy and is called the Centro Studi Martha Harris.

These training centers take people from various professions: usually child psychiatry, psychology, social work or education who wish to train to work psychoanalytically with children. In some cases, we had pediatricians or gynecologists or neurologists who wanted to find out more about psychoanalysis and psychoanalytic psychotherapy. There have been years when magistrates from juvenile court have attended the Centro Studi Martha Harris.

Martha Harris, a psychoanalyst for the British Psychoanalytic Society, influenced the development of the program. She structured the initial part of the program as a preliminary program to gather the interest of professionals in psychoanalytic principles. It was called an Observation Course in which two of the most important components were the Infant observation method of learning initiated by Esther Bick and the Work Discussion group. There was also a theoretical component but most of the course was experiential and meant to provide a setting in which "learning from experience" was

DOI: 10.4324/9781003167679-3

facilitated. Martha Harris was a student of Bion. His ideas inspired Martha Harris's construction of this method for learning that was unusual for psychoanalytic institutes at the time. Theory was relegated to a secondary position to learning from emotional immersion in observation of a family and a newborn baby for two years, and a work discussion seminar which was meant to encourage thinking about the relationship in work from psychoanalytic perspectives. It was thought that the theory would be understood through your experience of clinical work and not the other way around. This was a very important element that was needed for the development of the analytic attitude and the capacity to think for oneself. The idea of doing infant observation at the same time as beginning to bring your work to be understood in a new model was a particularly powerful combination of opening the student's perceptions and softening their psyches to emotional vibrations within themselves and others. As one can imagine, anxieties are aroused in the individuals and the group. The leaders of these two group experiences have to be skilled in containing the feelings and projections. The teachers work with the same group of students for the two years of their preclinical training. I think this consistency and depth really matters. Most of the students are in analysis or intensive psychoanalytic psychotherapy during this pre-clinical part of the course. The pre-clinical course includes reading Freud's clinical papers and important theory papers and then a year of reading Klein's papers. There is also a child development component that links psychoanalysis to developmental theories and research.

Mrs. Bick's extraordinary discovery of the use of infant observation to begin the task of growing within the individual a place to observe and reflect on one's own emotions aroused by observing an infant with his mother and father in the first years of life. This intimate and vulnerable time in a family and the needs of the infant and mother challenges the student's ability to take in this complex time and respond in a way that allows the student to continue to observe. With the help of the seminar leader and the group which act as a container to process the experience, the student internalizes this thinking space which facilitates the student's ability to see more clearly what the infant and the parents may be feeling. As one can see, this is clearly an analytic model of learning, as it were, with the help of your objects. Moreover, it helps you to work with emotional situations with heightened projections utilizing your counter-transference as a compass.

Through the years of teaching students in this program and many others here in New York with this Tavistock method of learning, I am struck and amazed how my students develop from not being able to imagine what another person might be thinking, to being able to form sensitive conjectures about a person's unconscious world. It is always informed by their ability to understand their own responses to their patient.

Many years ago, I had an extraordinary paper presented to me among others at the end of the two-year course. It was a paper written by a young pediatrician who was inspired by his work in pediatrics. The enlightened practitioner who worked in the progressive Prato (a small town in Italy) medical service desired to expand his own understanding by seeking first a Balint group and then a child psychoanalytic training. It was in his first two years of the pre-clinical observation course that I encountered Dr. Valentino Ammannati in a work discussion group that I lead. His struggles to put together his professional medical model and way of working with the new psychoanalytic model that he eagerly wished to acquire brought me in touch with the struggles that all medical practitioners including psychiatrists must need to confront and deal with in the process of learning. For this reason, I wish to share this remarkable paper with you as I think his paper describes a process of learning that I cannot imagine conveying more clearly. We present here only two of the three clinical cases in the paper.

Two Cases (by Valentino Ammannati)

Case I

I work as a "basic pediatrician" (but I prefer to call myself a family pediatrician) for the National Health Service in a local health unit of the district of Prato, a populous industrial city near Florence. I specialized in Pediatrics at the University of Florence in 1982. Since then, I have been working almost exclusively as a pediatrician. At first, I also worked at the hospital, but later only as a family pediatrician. For many years I have been following about 800 children (500 families) of an age ranging from birth to 14 years. We have manifold and global functions, established by a national convention, not just the diagnosis and cure of the pathologies in the outpatient's department and at home.

We also focus on health, education, prevention, and all that is needed to help the child and his family to reach and maintain his psycho-physical health in its widest meaning. This is therefore a truly important role, implying huge responsibility, but it is also extremely gratifying. In reality, as long as I studied at the university, both for the degree in medicine and during the specialization in pediatrics, this "global approach" to the "cure" (also viewed as "taking care of the patient") has never been taught to us. The prevailing view of our profession was mainly mechanistic, based on an organic explanation.

Thus, when I began to work, the relational aspects of children with their families came unexpectedly to be part of my work, and I found myself completely unprepared. I often felt the distress of experiencing situations which were emotionally richer and full of strong projections that I was not able to understand. I did not know what was happening to me and why. I was not even able to understand the questions, which were often confused, insistent, sometimes unexpressed; the parents asked questions concealing the distress, the pain which I painfully felt but I could not give a real answer to, whenever I wrote a "prescription" or "gave some advice." It was because of this distress that I felt intuitively there was something else that I did not understand and that I did not know, with regard to both my little patients and myself. So, together with a group of pediatricians, who shared my anxieties, we decided to organize a Balint group led by two psychoanalysts.

It was the year 1987, and it had taken me five years to find this first path. As I was used to reason following the rules of protocols, I hoped I would learn to "protocol feelings," to understand readily the problem at stake, to interpret and give a satisfactory answer. I hoped that all of this would also be reached quickly not to interfere much with my working schedule as "basic pediatrician," and that I would soon free myself from the anxiety of not understanding everything immediately. My being able to give immediate answers seemed vital. However, the experience of the Balint group, which helped me see the strength and the complexity of my feelings which emerged, led me to decide to begin a personal analysis, which gave me the possibility to begin to understand better what was happening to me. I thought it would also help me in my rapport with the children and their families.

This is how I got to the Tavistock Observation Course: I was looking to find a way to feel more satisfied with my work and maybe (citing Winnicott) also because "the psychoanalytic research has always been, to some extent, an attempt on the part of the analyst (pediatrician) to push the work of his own analysis beyond the limit that his analyst helped him reach."

I found myself in a Work Discussion Group the first year of the Observation Course. The first "case" that I brought to the group was that of David, a 17-month-old only child. No "big problem," only many questions on the part of the parents, who expressed worries and uncertainties that made me perceive some distress. It was because, of this distress that the parents kept looking for an answer, although still within the ambit of the "normal" check-ups.

Now I think I chose this case also because it was a good example, for its "normality," of a common situation that pediatricians often have to face: while the doctor is gathering "objective" data, the parents start talking of their doubts, their anxieties, and pains in the relationship with their child.

As I re-read my report, I realize that since the beginning I felt the need to describe the type of "setting" of a pediatric unit: the unexpected visits, the lack of time, the anxiety when I felt the urge to find adequate answers for everybody. The group gave me the understanding and the solidarity that I needed to face my difficulty in performing a good listening function. There was also rage for the sense of fatigue I felt in taking care of the difficult aspects of my work and that nobody had taught me to face during the course at the university. Rage for feeling like I was torn between two sides: the organic and the psychological. It was as if I had to fight at the same time on two opposite sides within a context where you cannot say no to anybody: to people who do not respect the time, to people requesting the consultations during the day, to the telephone calls in the out-patient department. The frustration in finding some time to think and do one thing at a time. There was also the rage due to the feeling that my time, with such indefinite limits, and my consultations (too many in a day), did not have any value. Along with this rage there was also the envy of my colleagues at the Tavistock Course, who in my opinion had the possibility of taking care of only one aspect of their patient. They met patients with more definite appointment times.

I immediately realized that these feelings were maybe only due to the suffering one feels when you start facing a crisis which leads you to finding a new role. How difficult it is to bear the idea of letting go of an old skin that we used to live in and to find another skin which will fit you better and will give you satisfaction. How scary the feeling is that we will not be able to find ourselves again, and to abandon our usual professional roles without knowing what you will become.

During the two years of the course I felt (and I still do) that I was looking for that integration which could allow me to go on, to feel better about myself; to maintain some continuity and integrity with my past history.

After the group discussion on the first meeting with David and his family it seemed to me I understood better some aspects which had seemed confusing. My feelings and my reactions and acting out the themes which emerged, were a means to think about the function that I could have performed in that situation. David's mother says that the child "is aggressive; he does not tolerate limitations, disobeys, he is more aggressive than others." Father and mother say "we do not know how to behave," although they try to understand him more by getting a wider view of David's life. I ask how and with whom he spends his days. I feel pushed to give immediate answers like doctors are used to do. In this case the answer was just words: words of understanding (from part of me also a parent): "At this age it is tiring and fatiguing to stay with children." The words then became a sort of brief conference based on an educational approach: "I understand that certain moments are difficult, one is tired and it seems that things are not changing whereas children grow and they continuously change, always providing us with new problems."

From the group, it emerged that my behavior was perhaps a way to deal with the projections of the parents and the expectations on me in the transference. It was like I had fallen into a trap: I did something defensively, to try to soothe and calm the anxiety of the parents and my own anxieties as well. Karen brings a thought that "Once you start doing things you stop thinking."

My anxiety pushed me to reassure. It did not allow me to recognize the anxiety of the mother, who continued to be worried. I had not listened to her. In fact, after the visit, I tell her "David has grown well." She answers: "It is a problem to make him eat." When she walks out, she lingers on the threshold to say one more thing: "David has some small blisters on his leg."

This last statement conveys to me that the mother is not heard and that my interventions are insufficient: while we talk, David is still agitated. The mother tries to keep him still. She has an absent look. She seems tired, exhausted, maybe disheartened.

What are the themes emerging from this meeting? How could I have made better use of the transference of David's mother that made me respond? The atmosphere of the visit also reflects the control of the father, as opposed to the anxiety and the sense of fatigue of the mother. David walks resolutely around the office, touching pieces of furniture and objects with the keys. David's passion for keys makes me think about the theme of going in and out of the maternal object. He may be afraid to stay inside, penetrating the object. He might damage it and then he must come out of it. But if he goes out he may be projected outwards and lose it: he does not feel good either inside or outside.

"We cannot make him have his hair cut," the father says. Hair cutting is a sort of growth ritual; maybe it is the mother who does not accept it: it would be like offering the baby to the father. This difficulty may be a problem of mother–child separation. Selecting these communications ripe with phantasy, I could have asked the parents to think about the things that each brought to me. I could have approached the father with the problem, so that he could be involved too. I could have facilitated the parents talking together. The father is not able to come into this relationship. He could facilitate the separation that the mother seems unable to tolerate. The father could contain the aggression that is inherent in separation and weaning.

The seminar leader brings a metaphor. The father has a regulatory function like a nipple between the breast and the child's mouth, otherwise there would be a continuous flow of milk out from the breast. The father performs this function for example in helping mother to see when her baby can wait. The father is also worried, but he reacts through control and denial. I began to understand the need for this paternal function; I could see more clearly my role of containing the mother's anxieties. I could make clear that she was worried, despite the fact that her child was perfectly healthy. I could help her differentiate the two realities: the healthy child and the child in her mind. I could work gradually on this awareness and perhaps propose a meeting with the mother alone. From this meeting, there could emerge a link between her worrying about her child and her own needs. The mother needed a recognition of her problems. The group helped me to formulate that one of the skills of the doctor is to facilitate thinking and exploring together. This is more difficult than giving prescriptions or interpretations.

In the second meeting which I brought to the group, there emerges the theme of my identification with David. During a home visit, I observe that "David does not have a bedroom of his own. In the room, there is a sofa bed, the television ... and a bed on wheels that at night is moved into the parent's bedroom." The parents still talk to me about the difficulties with the child.

The father says that "David is more tranquil with the grandparents. On Friday, when the mother comes, he gets agitated, and on Saturday, when I arrive, he becomes restive. It is his mother's fault and also mine ... Maybe we give in too much with him!" "Maybe we make him go out too much," the mother says. "Maybe he goes out too little," the father says.

I felt that David was lonely and lost in this confusion. The father added: "We'd do anything for him, we kill ourselves to take him out and make him enjoy himself. If he does not go out he becomes crazy: he wants to go out all the time." I replied, "It seems that he does not like to stay home." Within myself, I thought that David did not feel good either with his father or with his mother. This feeling certainly increased the defensiveness of the parents.

Karen suggests: "Each time you think: these parents do not understand their child you are in a difficult position. You are only looking at one point of view." The capacity to identify with both the child but also with the parents makes it possible to understand the family situation.

Splitting can trigger guilt and therefore defenses. In this respect, I felt my difficulty to fight against a mental attitude which tried to lay the blame on somebody (in this case on both parents). I understood that to blame somebody is a way to defend myself from the anxiety of a situation causing pain: I identified with David and I found myself ready to hurl myself against these "unfit" parents who did not understand him. Furthermore, it was a way to remove the feeling of my own incapacity and helplessness with the situation. I felt the same difficulties in my experiences with the infant and young child observation that I was doing at the time of this seminar.

When the mother goes out to work and hands David (she was holding him in her arms) to his father, I noticed that neither the father nor the mother talk to him. David cries desperately and afterwards I ask the father if he talks to David; if he explains to him what is happening. The father answers that he does not. I realized that this inquiring attitude makes the father feel guilty. With the help of the group I understood that instead of asking a question, I could have given voice to thoughts, to the feelings of the father, saying: "It must be difficult to talk to David when he acts like this. How difficult it is to hear him cry without knowing why." To offer a response as a "thinking model" may help the parents to think without making them feel guilty.

The seminar leader brings us the thought of Bion: "Thinking is different than having thoughts." To think, it is necessary to have some space. The original emotional space is created by the mother, who does not "know" but offers a thinking model as she wants to understand. Maybe in this case the parents do not have this model of an internal mother who allows them to think, a model to facilitate thinking, and thinking together. My function could be to supply them with a space, with a model to facilitate thinking on how to think about their child. Maybe this need is expressed by the mother when she walks out of the house while David is crying. She waves goodbye to

David from the threshold of the open door. She waves goodbye to me and then runs away. This response seems to have an infantile emotional response, as she waves me goodbye like a child to her "pediatrician–mother."

Another important aspect which emerges from the group discussion is the possibility of David's father being jealous. It seems that the mother identifies with the child. The father does not. Therefore, he is in a difficult position both in respect to the couple, wife–son and to me. This could activate feelings of rivalry and envy toward me. When I invite him for a meeting together with his wife at the outpatient's department, because "they seemed in a critical situation," he answers that "there are problems with the time." Maybe, it could have been a relief for the father to know that I understood his pressure and that I shared with him my not knowing. To admit not to know is fatiguing but may help to create a space for thinking: it is difficult to put this together with the role of the doctor. It would have been a relief to make him know that I understood the conflict with his wife, saying: "How difficult it is to have different opinions and to find points of agreements, seeing that the child needs both of you."

Case 2

In the work discussion group, I also chose to present the case of Melania, who suffers from recurrent pains to her legs, because it represented another typical situation for pediatricians. I found myself in the presence of a form of distress that required first to establish whether it had an organic basis or whether it was "functional." This is the term they taught me to use at the university for the definition of some forms of distress that could be important and sources of pain, but that could not be classified among the organic illnesses. In the Department of Internal Medicine, which I attended during the years of the university, when you came across a case where you had to exclude an organic illness, even the most prepared doctors "settled the question" by talking of some functional distress. This was considered the area for psychiatrists or psychologists. As I was writing, I realized that it is difficult to come out of this dualism. I must say that doctors always think in terms of the threat of wrong diagnoses of "functional" problems. The term "psychosomatic" has reached the academic world more recently, with years of delay due to the resistance to recognize the possibility that psychic suffering may manifest itself with physical problems and illnesses and also beyond the strict limits of the psychiatric illnesses. Presently, following the new and more sophisticated tests which have shown the close connection between chemical neuro-mediators and disturbances which once were thought as *"sine substantia"* (these tests have proven and measured with the use of neuro-radiological surveys which once were not possible, that there are metabolic and circulatory changes linked to behavioral distress), I believe that one of the reasons why I began studying medicine was to answer the question: "Why does one get sick?" This question perhaps hides another question: "Why does one suffer?" The case of Melania once more proposed these questions.

It seems to me that during the meeting with the parents I was able to use my awareness as it emerged in the group discussion, helped in this by my previous reports and by the observations of all the other members of the group. It was as if I could finally begin to think without acting, that I could think together with the parents without forgetting my role as doctor: "After having examined the X-rays and the check-ups for a complete clinical evaluation, I confirm that there are no changes." I begin to talk, saying: "I would like to hear from each one of you what you think of Melania's problem, what is the idea that you have made of it." I was also able to admit that I did not know what might have been the original cause of the pains in Melania's legs and I invited them to talk together to see if we could understand more about the problem. It seems to me that Melania's parents and I have been able to create a space and a time to think together without feelings of guilt or of judgements, preconceptions that would have hindered our research.

There emerged, from the parents, a series of themes which may constitute the basis for thinking and searching into the causes of Melania's problem. The father says: "When she feels the pains she wants to be cuddled by her mother, she sends me away and then she gets desperate and says: 'I do not want to grow.' Why does she say this to me? She says this because she heard that these pains are growth pains." "As if it was painful to grow?" I observe. Mother:

> Since she had the measles, she did not want to go back to bed anymore. In any case, she makes us feel guilty, she says that it is not right that we should sleep together and she by herself. She is jealous. She wants things at all costs. She is stubborn and tells me that I am bad. It has been so since she went to the kindergarten. Before it was different. I gave her a lot of caring and attention, she may have felt that she missed me. Lately, we had some worries too because we changed houses. When we went to see the new house she was sad and said: We won't move here, will we?

I say to them, "It seems that separations, first from the mother then from the house, cause her problems." Mother: "Yes, I think so." I comment, "On the other hand, parents are worried about Melania's pains." The mother asks: "What do we have to do? How do we have to behave?" I am not able to give an answer to these questions. Instead I propose: "We could talk again, if you felt the need to," revealing my feeling that they needed more space to think. If I offer them more time to talk and meet, my hope is that the parents will expect to talk of their mental problems and pains. The group made me aware how my offer connected to their unconscious needs, and it seemed that I was in touch with the parents, which in turn made them more open to unconsciously taking in the need of their child.

Through the group and the leader, I understood that it is this that helps to connect to the psychosomatic illnesses; the elaboration of the meaning of physical pain and transferring it on the mental plane. In the discussion of this case, I brought to the group all of my doubts and the confusion about the limits of my role as pediatrician. My questions were many and full of anxiety: what are my functions as pediatrician? What are my limits? To propose new meetings to these parents means to go into a field which does not belong to me?

I remember very well the seminar leader's response, that this is my conflict. The parents believe they can get the help they need from me. The therapeutic role which I may perform, without doing psychotherapy (with occasional meetings or brief series of meetings) is a containing role. To supply a space which contains through observing and responding. Is this not what I try to learn in this course: offering the parents the tools to think?

In the next meeting with Melania's mother, I hid a tape recorder, which I started at the beginning of the interview. Why? What I told myself before was that I wished to report to the group a work situation that guaranteed objectivity. I even imagined hiding a video camera. I was afraid that my memory may alter the situation and the dialogues. Maybe as someone in the group made me aware, it was also a way to feel less stress due to the effort of remembering and rewriting the meeting which was what we were meant to do for our presentations. This new "discovery" came right in the moment when I began to perceive a little more clearly how my role of doctor could change and improve, and which were the more complete functions that I could learn to perform. Was this "recording" a kind of regression to some previous position? To record is a little like measuring: to give objectivity also to emotions which are aroused during a meeting. It was a way to reconfirm my belonging to a "scientific thought," which works on reliable data, and that can be reproduced. Was it a way to give voice to the doubts, which I often have about the scientific aspect of psychoanalysis? Was it a way to keep me away from my emotions? Perhaps too many for my capacity to stand them and welcome them?

Melania's mother arrives suddenly at the outpatient department asking for a medicine for Melania's pains in her legs. "It is not a psychological problem," she says at the beginning. From the interview that follows there emerge important aspects of her relationship with her child: Melania's jealousy toward the father, her wanting to be at the center of attention, the greed to have everything, the fatigue of the mother. "We no longer have our space. We do not go out anymore, we go out for her." I am told the story of what happens when Melania has her fits which leads the mother to talk of her own childhood experiences.

It is at this point that I try to link the pain in Melania's legs. I say, "It seems that this pain in her legs allows her to have specific things, like these stories [about her own childhood] ... and that it gives her the chance to give voice to the feelings which makes her feel guilty." Melania seems insatiable to the mother. The mother also knows that medicines do not heal: "I see that it is enough that I give her some attention even for two minutes and she is totally happy." But she cannot stand the sense of guilt toward the daughter. In prescribing the drug for the pain at the end of the meeting I seem to share, with the mother, the sense of guilt for Melania's pain: she feels like this because she would like "to give her everything" but she does not do it. I too feel that continuing the meetings could be of help, but I do not feel like doing it. The mother seems to want to say: "What else may I do for Melania in addition to buying her everything? And not to sleep with my husband anymore, almost?" She feels deprived by the child. She would like to be available but she cannot respond any longer. I could have shared with her the uncertainty of not knowing what to do. I could have expressed an understanding of her exhaustion and understand that she needs someone with whom to share all this. I could have asked her if it was the need of a drug, or if she really thought there was a need for us to talk about this again, leaving the decision to her. I could have also helped the mother to say no to the child sometimes. I could suggest that there was no need to come for the drug. She could come there just to talk and that talking seemed to help her.

I think that my availability toward the mother of Melania was limited. How can I be available for all the patients (they are about 500 families)? Maybe it is for this reason that I prescribed the drug at the end; looking for some short cut, perhaps identified with "feeling unfit as a mother." I too shared with mother the sense of helplessness and limitation at not coming up with an answer or solution. With this work, I tried to pull the threads together of the Intense impact of the work discussion group in these last two years. What I could understand and "fix" in this final report depends mostly on the work done in the group: an experience of active and affective learning in which the emotional parts are at play rather than theoretical knowledge in the relationship with our patients.

As I was thinking about the cases, I could not avoid thinking about my own history, about the choices that I have gradually made as I gained awareness that the therapeutic role of the doctor should not be identified and does not end with the interpretation of "objective" data which emerged from a medical test. It is not just a diagnosis or a drug prescription or providing advice. It is, without a doubt, something much more complex and variegated. Inevitably, my doubts, my anxieties, my incapacities emerged in the discussion and in the elaboration of the cases. It seems to me that I was able to see them a little more clearly, gathering from it a better comprehension of my feelings in the relationship with my patients and their suffering.

My oscillating. between an organic view and a psychodynamic approach, toward illnesses and suffering echoed with yet other oscillations: the omnipotence of the medical role and the frustration in the contact with my patients and myself when I had to face the reality of my difficulties in taking care of others; the oscillations between idealization and denigration; hate and love between me and my patients. Finally, the oscillation between the choice to continue being a pediatrician and to start a formation path as a child psychotherapist.

I still feel that I am looking for an integration among these various aspects, although it seems to me that the experience of these last two years gave me the possibility to see things more clearly, maybe because I suspended that mental attitude of judgement and activated the capacity of getting used to uncertainty. We all shared these experiences during the observations and in the work discussions.

Commentary (by Karen Proner)

Dr. Ammannati did return to pediatrics, where he is still practicing fifteen years later. He has said that this was a very important experience for him that has influenced his work in pediatrics.

As I look at this paper, it is clear that this way of working with other professionals is a very powerful way of introducing psychoanalytic thinking and skills to our colleagues who may continue to practice in their own professional roles. It contains uncertainties and anxieties that they already feel and struggle with. If their anxieties are contained it can deepen and enhance their experiences with their patients.

Chapter 3

On Becoming a Parent
When the Psychoanalyst Meets the Front-Line Professionals Involved in the Perinatal Period

Meropi Michaleli

Introduction

J. Raphael-Leff (1993), a pioneer in the theoretical and clinical comprehension and therapeutic techniques in psychoanalytic work with pregnant women, was courageous enough to state that the yardstick for a civilized country is shaped by the measures and care practices contemplated and applied for the protection of the health of pregnant women and newly born infants.

This is what has shaped the basis, while rising to become the central theoretical reference, in our work. On our part, we endeavored to examine the existing framework of perinatal and postnatal interventions in Greece. What is the environment of psychic care and assistance pregnant women may expect to benefit from during their pregnancy and the postnatal period? And what are the services an expecting couple can refer to before they come to us psychoanalysts/therapists, when in a state of despair?

It is with deep dismay that we have realized that the public health structures capable of providing comprehensive services of mental assistance and psychopathological prevention during the perinatal period are almost non-existent, while the rest of available modules are understaffed, struggling to meet the increasing needs for health and wellbeing services.

Pre- and Postnatal Psychopathology

It is a well-known fact that the major issues in the field of mental health of our times, both in this country and throughout the European Union, are maternal depression, and more specifically the manifestations of depression experienced during the perinatal period (from pregnancy until the 12th month of out-of-womb life).

Pregnancy and motherhood have always been seen as a period of happiness during which the woman feels fulfilled and is immune to psychiatric disorders. While pregnancy is a period of joy and fulfillment for many women, there are studies revealing an increase of psychiatric disorders and, depression during pregnancy (Karmaliani et al., 2009). According to the WHO, by 2020 depression will be the second cause of death in the world after heart diseases. Moreover, epidemiological studies have shown that women are bound to suffer twice as much from depression compared to men, with the reproductive period seen as a high-risk period (Meltzer-Brody, 2011).

According to international and Greek statistical data, depression is, unlike postnatal psychosis which is tantamount to 1.5 ‰, far more common, even though only 50% of the cases are diagnosed and only 18% receive treatment. During pregnancy, 15–20% of women will manifest minor or major postnatal depression and 10–15% of mothers will do so from labor onwards until the 12th month of the out-of-womb life (Bennett et al., 2004; Faisal-Cury et al., 2007; Teixeira et al., 2009). International literature reports that major risk factors include depression during pregnancy (by 70%), high prenatal stress (by 41%), medical history of mental disorder, poor support network and social isolation, and other critically stressful life events (mourning, immigration, break-up, unemployment).

Maternal psychopathology is a leading cause of maternal mortality, second only to gynecological complications during pregnancy and labor. Depression during the perinatal period impacts the mother, the infant and the family at all levels. Consequently, prevention, early detection and treatment of perinatal depression in the mother is a major issue of public health promotion that concerns both the mother herself, and the child as well as the broader family and social context (Salomonson, 2018). Maternal depression increases cost at the level of mental health services and at public hospitals (Bauer et al., 2014) as it is related to:

- **The difficulty or incapacity of the mother to take care of her baby**, as she is herself often in need of mental health care and has to give up custody of the child to day-care institutions, foster families and other providers of mental health services.
- **A small for dates (lower birth weight) and increased prematurity** necessitating hospitalization in neonatal intensive care units where there is need for long-term medical and psychological support, due to the range of regulatory disorders and developmental problems prematurity may cause: high levels of cortisol, resulting in high irritability and difficult consolability, sleep and food disorders, early attachment disorders, autism, epilepsy, neurological problems and, later on, learning difficulties (Goodman, 2007). Under such circumstances, the cost of necessary services (medical, psychiatric, educational, specialized accommodation facilities and day care centers) is really high as it is bound to span over an extended period of time.
- **Infant abuse cases.** This significantly impacts an infant's development and may lead to extreme behaviors in adult life, such as delinquency and

substance abuse, which socially and economically burden the wellbeing state.
- **Infant mortality**, entailing psychological and financial costs for the community. Greece used to have one of the lowest percentages of infantile mortality in Europe. This has dramatically changed over the last five years, as in times of peace, the Greek index of infantile mortality has increased from 10‰ to 40‰. Such unprecedented increase in figures in this domain is only expected in countries at war. The rise of the infantile mortality rate mirrors the consequences of the socioeconomic crisis affecting Greece. It has been historically proven that infants are more vulnerable to the consequences of a generalized socio-economic crisis, which is manifested by the increase of infantile mortality, as stated above (Parsons et al., 2012).

Another new major issue of public health has been the large influx of immigrants over the last 5 years. Immigration implies loss, separation from the maternal figure and the affiliated family; the birth process, as a whole, rekindles the need to revisit the maternal representation. Therefore, these women are expected to identify with the traditional maternal representation and function, while cut off from every point of external maternal figure of reference. They are away from their culture and traditions, far from their own mother and support network, while also having to adapt to a new homeland, which is not always a "nurturing embrace." The birth of children to first generation immigrants, people abruptly cut off from their roots, their homeland, their language and their civilization, entails a multiple bereavement and loss process that such people find neither the space nor the time to express, let alone experience with the assistance of health professionals in the host country. In those cases when immigrant parents during the pregnancy and the birth of their child are psychologically supported by perinatal and neonatal professionals in the host country, they are offered an opportunity that allows them to experience a feeling of continuity of their existence, despite the successive severances and losses they have been suffering.

A Psychoanalyst in the Neonatal Intensive Care Unit

It is really all about the way the psychoanalyst is meant to liaise with professionals of the perinatal team and more specifically within the context of neonatal intensive care units. As a matter of fact, the idea of a clinic dedicated to premature births and the prolonged care necessary for the period to follow, has for some time now been high on our agenda – and increasingly so it is bound to remain, all the more since, over the last 20 years, more and more labors originate from medically assisted procreation. Such births are happening under circumstances that leave parents, the neonate as well as the healthcare staff, rather vulnerable. In such cases, us Psychoanalysts are, together with all other members of the perinatal care unit, called upon to consider whether and under what conditions, there may be discussion about the psychical meaning to the day-to-day care practices developed in "emergency mode," in such clinics. Moreover, we should consider how us psychoanalysts could, along with the rest of members on the team, reduce the influence of morbid factors affecting the dyad mother-infant or the triad mother-father-infant.

Clinical Vignette

I want you to show me where it is I was born ...

Those are the first words Yianni, age 6, at the time, addressed to me upon entering the neonatal intensive care unit that morning, as part of a follow-up routine he had been admitted for. He nevertheless knew that that was not where he had been born; rather, his birth had taken place in a maternity clinic, other than the pediatric hospital where we now stood. Still, in so telling me, he may just as well have been expressing the crux of the issue herein discussed, albeit in his own, special way:

To their parents, premature infants "are born twice." It is as if two dates of birth are transcribed in the parents' memory and so they are transmitted to them through the parental experience: the first, "traumatic" date of birth is the one occurring on the day when the intra-uterine life is discontinued before completion. Otherwise said, this is about neonates/fetuses having to complete their intra-uterine development in an extra-uterine environment. Such first birth happens in the maternity ward, within a context of emergency, with medical technology getting from the onset the upper hand in a process that was once known and familiar to us, as it followed "the nature's path." Premature birth implies a threat to the survival of the infant and sometimes to that of the mother. The second date of birth is the one considered by the parents to be their baby's actual biological arrival: this is the day when they may actually take their infant away from the neonate intensive care unit, home with them, after a hospitalization having lasted anything from a couple of weeks to several months. More often than not, when asked about their baby's birthday, parents are bound to get confused between such two dates.

Yianni was born in the 28th week of gestation. He had to stay in the Neonatal Intensive Care Unit for three months, six weeks of which he spent under mechanical ventilation.

On the day scheduled for the interview, Yianni came dressed in a way very much reminiscent of a "business executive": jacket, long trousers, round spectacles. The way he moved, the expressions on his face, his gestures and the whole posture of his, left something to be desired, as if everything about him was cramped and foreign. He sat down and started scribbling out a sketch typical, development-wise, of a 3-year-old child. Emotional atonia, kinetic inertia, limited interaction and communication/psychosomatic vulnerability, are the main diagnostic signs of an early child depression, all of which had been present in Yianni's case. At the beginning of the interview, the mother stated that from the day her son was born, she has never been away from him a single moment, be it day or night. They even share the same bed. The first-time mother and son were apart was when, at the age of 5 and a half, the boy was enrolled at the nursery school. As soon as he left home, he developed what his mother calls a "paroxysmic cough," eventually diagnosed by the MD as asthma. As coughing persisted to the point of Yianni vomiting, his mother eventually had him leave the nursery school.

"I cannot take it anymore, I am done," the exasperated mother told me. "I am on it at all times, I am so stressed about Yianni and his state of health." I replied: "It is as if you were a hostage under such concerns and worries you have about Yianni – you cannot get away from them."

I then turned to Yianni: "Yianni, how does it feel, today with you and mom coming to visit us?"

(May I stress, at this point, that Yianni and his mother had checked in at the Neonatal Intensive Care Unit earlier than scheduled. She herself actually asked the head nurse to let them in and be guided around the place where "he was born").

To which question, without hesitation or second thoughts Yianni responded:

YIANNI: I wanted to go goo-goo, again! [Pause]
ANALYST: Go goo-goo again?
YIANNI: Sure, [go back to] that time when I had little tubes into my nose and syringes and mom used to come to me as I woke up and gave me the dummy!!

Early Bonding between Yianni and His Mother

Just as the case is for any relationship between a prematurely born infant and its mother, Yianni was at birth forthwith deprived of the gratification an infant and its mother are bound to share, both during breast-feeding and at the time of prime care. The day care has, in this case, been undertaken by the medical and nursing staff. Hence a contradiction: on one hand there is a privation of gratifications originating from the primal relationship between the mother and thew new-born, whereas on the other there occurs an obstruction of the capacity of autoregulation, otherwise present in born term infants.

In the case of premature infants, the pare-excitation function of the mother is from the onset deactivated. On the other hand, the mother and the new-born infant are exposed to a flow of a plethora of perceptual stimuli and arousals originating from the medical/ technological context which, with such interventions, embarks upon an effort to save the infant. Obviously, the mother/ parents are not given the opportunity of airing their envy and aggressiveness vis-à-vis this team set out to save their child's life, when they were unable to carry out the task of safeguarding and completing intrauterine life.

How does the sense of the parents' security, with respect to the efficacy of services offered to their offspring, affect the progress of the infant's health while in hospital care?

Yianni's vital functions, especially that of respiration, had for a long period of time being threatened. Such threat to his life was, amongst other, also maintained through the mother's overstimulation. Her ongoing presence next to Yianni, day and night, had been something of an enhancer to the infant's mechanical respiratory support, for as long as such mechanical support was on, until she took over, upon disconnection of the ventilator. The mother's physical presence had been as overwhelming and continuous as that of Yianni's ventilator.

This clinical vignette presented, makes one wonder how differently things could have developed, if the perinatal team that assisted that dyad had timely comprehended the early indication of disorders present in the primary relationship between the mother and the prematurely born infant and in the emerging mental life. How could such knowledge eventually help shape the way parents are assisted by the staff? How can practices of such staff be influenced towards helping mitigate primal death stress in the mother, against which the latter eventually struggled by insisting on a relentless physical presence by Yianni and by feeling unable to let go of the child?

Psychodynamic Interventions in Pregnancy and during the Perinatal Period

Any early prevention program on the perinatal and infantile period, aimed to prevent psychopathology in the newborn/infant and/or to avert the repetition of a transgenerational pathology in new parents, is based on two assumptions. First, during the process of transition to parenthood, early parental caregiving and the quality of the primary experiences are encoded in the body, the brain and the psyche of the embryo/newborn, contributing to their shaping and structuring. Such premise implies that, in order to interrupt the process of repetition and the transmission of intergenerational trauma infiltrating from the very beginning the mother–fetus/newborn relationship, early interventions have to be established already at pregnancy.

Through the messages and the meanings which are created in the primary body-to-body, the two members of the dyad become acquainted with the rhythmic pace of one another and will modify their behaviors so as to adapt to this flow, co-creating in this way, (conditional on everything developing normally), a harmonious communication. Through these primary messages that use the body as a channel of transmission, the early relationship as well as the security it provides will be assessed. The need for security will always carry the trace of the initial backdrop, even when it will rid itself off of the early somatic forms in the course of time. It is important to note that the establishment of the early interaction between the mother and the infant is largely due to the fact that there is a particularity in the psychic function of the pregnant woman/ mother-to-be. Bydlowski (1991) named this "psychic transparency" (in French: *transparence psychique de la grossesse*) and Raphael-Leff (1993) "unconscious permeability." An important restructuring of the psychic structures takes place in the pregnant woman/ new mother: repressed memories and representations or even unrepresented states of mind, in the sense that the mother had been unable to represent them, giving them a meaning of her own. The return of the once "infantile" is dominant in the mother's internal world. The representations of the child-to-be born are non-existent or poor. The access to material, which was until then repressed or non-represented (whereas stored in the mother's implicit memory), will allow her to release the emotions associated with these experiences and invest this energy in her child so that she can adapt to its needs. We may therefore see that access to parenthood has been in the works since the early inscriptions of parental care experiences, which the parent herself received as a newborn. Neuron circuits created at that time, will be activated and determine the way in which the person will organize the relationship with the newborn as a parent (Mayes, 2005). In light of the above considerations, the therapeutic interventions are more effective when they begin during pregnancy. When negative experiences of early parental care are dominant, the therapeutic interventions after birth or even during the first months of the newborn's life already allow for the repetition of the traumatic circuit to be activated. The reversal/transformation of an established pathology both on the physical as well as on the psychic level is not to be taken for granted.

Second, the professionals working on that period of life, those who literally work on the "body- to-body" of the future mother and the embryo-newborn, are the first ones to welcome the parents' concerns, the infant's but also their own, whenever they are asked to work together. What we frequently see in new parents who come to see us in despair, is that many of early traumas that occurred at their baby's birth and further on, during the process of accessing parenthood, are related with projections they received from the therapists themselves who worked with them and contained them during the period of pregnancy, birth and the perinatal period.

An ever-increasing number of births occur after medically assisted reproduction. In some other cases, birth is followed by a long-term mechanical support of the newborn, due to its great prematurity and therefore, a long-term stay in the intensive care unit is needed, away from the family environment. This is the way many of our young patients – young children or teenagers who we already see in our clinical practice came to life. In cases of newborns and infants facing life-threatening conditions, parents should be assisted by a multidisciplinary team with specialized skills, familiar with the psychodynamic approach of the perinatal period and the processes taking place in the triad of the mother/mother-to-be, father-embryo/newborn, at a psychosomatic level. Infant, toddler and child therapists should have a comprehensive image of the evolving processes both at the body level as well as at the psychological level, during that phase. The existence of a network of front-line health professionals communicating and working towards a common goal around the parents-to-be/new parents, may ensure cohesion and continuity in their interventions, from the pre- through to the post-natal period, thus limiting the confusion of roles and the positions. Interventions of this nature should be expected to contribute to the reduction of confusion between the mother-father and newborn. In this way, a framework of emotional security is created for the parents and healthy parental identifications are activated, which is not the case when every involved specialist works on one's own, thus providing the family with fragmented health services. Often, the sense of discontinuity experienced by the parents of a hospitalized newborn along with the limbo such parents often feel they are in, is exacerbated by the incoherence/discontinuity of the practices of the perinatal health professionals. From the moment meetings with front-line health professionals take place in a coordinated way – creating a context within which parents are encouraged to express their feelings regarding the care and survival concerns of their infant or their inability to assume the parental role – then what is proposed to them by the collaborating perinatal team is a new "relationship model," which they will be asked to apply vis-à-vis their newborn. This intervention model by front-line health professionals is a "reparative experience" for the parents, a true epigenetic change, both in terms of their resilience to negative experiences and in terms of the possibility to internalize a positive parental relationship. A model of positive interactions is transferred unto them, which is different from the negative models of interaction of their childhood which overshadow the establishment of their relationship with their newborn infant. This constitutes an intervention against the repetition of transgenerational pathology. Access to parenthood is neither something granted, nor does it come free from obstacles, setbacks and ghosts from the past being present in the nursery. Becoming a parent can be a co-creation with the participation of three actors each one with its own contribution, which is affected and shaped by the other two while affecting them, shaping them and transforming them:

- **the newborn**, with its complex, rich, fragile and incomplete potential;
- **the parents** with their personal history, their expectations and their particularities; and

- **the therapists of the early intervention and** the perinatal team, who, by way of integrated practices around the infant and its family, may allow the parents a new transcription of their early care traumatic experiences.

The Program

In light of the above considerations, our project was based on a model of early care/intervention during the perinatal period developed and implemented both at the educational as well as at the clinical level, within a Public Maternity Hospital in Athens. These primary interventions were offered to professionals and families who would have otherwise not been able to access mental health services, where psychoanalytic thinking and understanding is at the very center of their design and implementation.

We embarked on this project asking ourselves two questions:

- What can a psychoanalyst contribute to this field?
- How can the psychoanalytical thinking be shared with healthcare personnel in perinatal services and the families they work with?

Our wish was that our contribution could hopefully, be two-fold. First, create awareness amongst professionals of disciplines other than psychoanalysis as well as instill in them the idea that our way of processing information when working with human beings, consists of thinking *before, during* and *after* we proceed to an act or practice. The staff working in pre- and post-natal settings usually strive towards getting control over their patients' bodily functions, by means of emergency medical and nursing practices without having the time to previously ponder about them.

Second, the potential realization that transition to parenthood is not given, but a co-creation involving parents, the newborn and the perinatal team working with them. This should involve the introduction and communication of a different way of thinking and understanding the beginning of the biological and mental life.

Our main theoretical references were the following:

- During the pre- and post-natal period, important transformations in the mother's mental function are taking place: memories repressed until then, find their way to consciousness, thus becoming accessible to re-elaboration (working through).
- During the process of transition to parenthood: early parental caregiving, and the quality of the initial attachment, are encoded in the body, the brain and the psyche of the embryo/newborn, contributing to their structuring. This means that the transition to parenthood "has been programmed" and shaped by the early experiences of parental caregiving, which the parents themselves had experienced: "We parent, as we have been parented."

The above imply that in order to interrupt the process of repetition and the transmission of intergenerational trauma infiltrating from the very beginning the mother–fetus/newborn relationship, a new model of relating with their baby has to be offered by perinatal front-line health professionals. When feeling contained and supported during pregnancy and at the time of birth of their baby, parents are offered a chance to experience a sense of continuity of their existence, despite previously experienced traumas and losses. A network of front-line health professionals (neonatologists, obstetricians, midwives, etc.) surrounding the family and working towards a common goal, may create an emotional security framework for parents, thus encouraging positive parental identifications.

The project was addressed to health care professionals from various disciplines (obstetricians-gynecologists, pediatricians, neonatologists, midwives, nurses, visiting nurses, social workers, psychologists and psychiatrists), who provide services to maternity and neonatal/ infant care settings in the public and private health sector throughout Greece.

The aim was raising awareness and providing training so persons in such disciplines may improve their skills in:

- recognizing the early signs/indications of maternal (and paternal) depression and reinforcing protective mechanisms against depression;
- recognizing early signs of repetition of parental pathology in the "here and now" of their establishing relationship; and
- enhancing the potential of establishment of a healthy and fulfilling parent–infant relationship.

Impact of the Project

Participants in the project (both professionals and parents) agreed that:

- In order to create a new shared knowledge and experience, a model of complementarity rather than substitution of the involved professionals is needed.
- The object of study and the interests of each professional object gains its meaning when in a dialectical exchange with other specialists' object of interest. In the case of perinatality, that means creating a space within which to think and care about the human being to be born and ultimately an identification with such being.
- The cohesion in communication between members of perinatal teams mitigates the confusion and fragmentation in their roles, positions and practices and consequently in the way such teams communicate with parents and baby which, in turn, contributes to reducing the role confusion among the mother, the father and the newborn baby.
- Besides, this model of interdisciplinary collaboration can lead to a decrease in professional burn-out and passive aggressive attitudes amongst colleagues as everyone shares the same goal and has more space

to think about the death anxiety and ambivalent feelings that are often overwhelming to them and the families.

What Professionals Attested

- The psychoanalytical understanding of the developing self provided professionals with a holistic view and understanding of physical as well as mental processes "at work" during this period. This constitutes for them a secure basis, as fragmentation, confusion and paralyzing projections in perinatal care can be reduced and even expunged.
- The professionals that participated and are still participating in this project, feel as if they have been offered a new, common language of communication and this way of thinking has been transferred to their professional contexts of origin.
- They feel safer and more confident in their practices, thus becoming more efficient with their infant patients and their families. They don't feel alone, isolated and frustrated any more, especially in a period when coherence is evading and substituted by aggression and violence, in our everyday lives. They now feel they belong to a wider network of people sharing similar ways of thinking and approaching the beginning of biological and mental life. Such co-created network protects them against their own omnipotence, emerging when they work on their own, believing that they "hold the truth," concerning a given family. It is for them a newly created space for reverie.

When asked to comment on the benefit of this project, the head midwife of the main Prenatal Care Department we have been working with stated the following:

> I feel not just lucky but blessed because, since the beginning of my career as a midwife I had the great opportunity of being part of the European Training Program for perinatal period health professionals, BIRTH AND FUTURE. Dr. Meropi Michaleli, psychoanalyst, was the specialist in charge of the scientific aspects of that program.
>
> I was emotionally touched, and I understood the nature of my profession. That program changed my attitude and helped me realize the real needs of the women and their babies. It was clear enough that I had found the way to treat the women and their babies with affection and understanding, without fear. I felt strong enough to face and give solutions to very provocative situations.
>
> Besides myself, my colleague midwives, nurses and everyone in the hospital started to face their job differently. The most amazing thing is that since 1996, health professionals that followed the program admit that their way of facing mothers and babies has been positively

influenced. We were affected not only professionally but even in our own lives as parents, couples, relatives or friends. It would not be an exaggeration to suggest that my life became more beautiful since that experience, I became a better person and a better midwife. I believe all women, babies and health professionals deserve this unique opportunity.

A video evaluation of the program, from the participants is available on YouTube (see https://www.youtube.com/watch?v=szQD3bQopik).

About the Parents

- As of antenatal and postnatal meetings, the discontinuity that the parents of a hospitalized new-born are likely to experience, may be reinforced by the discontinuity of actions and practices of the involved health professionals.
- Conversely, a holistic view and understanding of physical as well as mental processes "at work" during this period offers parents a space to express their anxieties concerning the survival of their newborn or their inability to take on their parental role, in an uncertain and rapidly evolving world. This is a new "relationship model" introduced by front-line therapists, which parents may identify with and apply in the relationship with their newborn. This new "relationship model" may hopefully lead to the internalization of positive parental qualities within their newly built relationship.
- This model of very early intervention constitutes a reparative experience for new parents, of the long-lasting kind for most of them; it is an epigenetic change to their resilience against intense and traumatic stimuli and experiences.

What We, as Psychoanalysts, Were Able to Convey through this Project to Our Colleagues Involved in Pregnancy and Post-Natal Period

There is an "unknown" in our body and mental function (in the sense of "unknown" mechanisms underlying fertility, infertility, the good state of health, or conversely, in the sickness of a newborn or premature baby). Our "unconscious" is being manifested to us only through the processes of its transformations. This acquired knowledge by the perinatal team professionals, is directly questioning the fantasies of omnipotence and control they can exercise over the mechanisms that govern somatic functions. Little by little, they become more familiar with this opening into the unknown, with the emptiness experienced by childless couples, or couples whose baby was born prematurely or ill, and did not return home with them. As far as we, psychoanalysts are concerned, the emptiness and the opening to the unknown, reminds us of what we experience when confronted with profound regressions in the transference/ countertransference.

In Greece, the perinatal care in the public sector is nonexistent, or at best very basic. Despite our efforts to put relevant modules in place over the last 20 years, there has been no structure in Greece to provide comprehensive services to sub-fertile couples, to mothers suffering from postnatal depression or to parents whose baby is born prematurely.

Our constant aspiration is to create further opportunities for such thinking spaces to be provided to professionals in public pre- and post-natal settings. I strongly believe that psychoanalysis has a lot to offer in this field. A psychoanalyst can work closely both with professionals in the perinatal teams (them being the recipients of strong parental projections and anxiety originating from parents and infants), and with the families themselves.

The latter is of paramount importance towards an early prevention of mental health problems. Through psychodynamic interventions during pregnancy, perinatal and early infant period, early parental traumas can be worked through, giving space for infant development to occur.

A Father

(Quotes the date), five minutes past Noon in Athens. Our daughter is born. This is the time after which the staff at the "Elena" [Maternity Hospital] helped me the most as a new father. For a week. My partner and I attended antenatal classes, which (despite being held in Greek, a language that I do not speak) helped me get in the mood of giving birth as a couple. Still, this can prepare a new father for what to expect after the baby is there with the parents. The staff at "Elena" were generally present, attentive and supportive but also discreet and most importantly emotionally available. They would teach you the intricate secrets of dealing with your baby needs without patronizing you. They would help you consider your baby as the real person she is and to allow yourself to really listen to her cries, receiving the tearing sounds as well as the voice of the baby that, as dirty and naked as she is, has just joined humanity without knowing that much about it. The staff at Elena won't provide you with a guide. They will be there supporting the most important survival activities the new father (the hero) is expected to carry out. Their presence is what counts, and it is exactly by being present with you to attend the new little person that the conditions for accepting the baby for what she is are created. It is hard work, though and there are a lot of ups and downs along the way. However, the memory of that experience is left within yourself as a beacon in the sky, and a man becomes a father by going back to it each and every time the route is lost.

A Mother

Deciding whether to give birth in London or in Athens had been really difficult for us. When we visited "Elena" and talked to the lead midwife as part of the decision-making process we felt really listened to and began to engage with our experience in a more real way. We discussed about our experience as an international couple, about the anxieties around birth and becoming parents in general, about the first few months after the baby's arrival. The connection I felt with this person was crucial in making up my mind. I found myself crying and crying. Was it that I spoke in Greek with a professional about my experience of becoming a mother after a long time? Was it something about the warmth of this woman and her willingness to listen to our story? Perhaps ... But thinking back I realize that in her presence I felt that my partner, who is Italian, had voiced important fears that I hadn't heard before. This was a great relief because his experience was attended by a professional in such an authentic way that freed me up and enabled me to stay with my own experience without needing to try and make space for him in processes that tend to be heavily focused on mothers. This experience was quite different from my experience of talking to professionals in London and other hospitals that we visited in Athens where I felt that people didn't have the time and energy to be curious about our experience.

Conclusions

A number of structures still remain latent, particularly those meant to ensure the mental and physical integrity of the person. In our daily work with extreme cases of pregnant women/women who have recently given birth and present a serious psychopathology, newborns and their families, a cooperation and a common line of thought by all the members of the medical team and the team of nurses is essential. Our concern, as Psychoanalysts, to share our knowledge on how the psyche works with the doctors of our body, obliges us to incorporate the various levels of a child's functioning in one single representation: the level of the body, psyche and emotion. Only then, what manifests itself as a somatic disorder in the infant or as a dysfunctionality in the early relationship can be understood as a psychic experience of the infant and the parents but also of the professionals. Without such cooperation, all clinical observations on newborns and infants are nothing but a list of behaviors.

In order to deepen and advance our knowledge regarding the conditions and the factors enhancing the physical and mental evolution of an infant, in particular when this infant is born under life-threatening conditions, pediatricians and psychoanalysts must move forward to join studies with mutual respect to our respective stances. Certainly, identifying and delimiting the various levels of the problem we have to face as professionals of different specialties, allows each one of us to find the place, the techniques and the methods used, as well as a way to conjugate them with those of the rest of the members of the team, through a perspective of complementarity rather than by substitution of one member by another. The issue of early subjective experiences and the interest in the early development of subjectivity does not simply concern the clinical praxis with young children. It concerns first and foremost the transmission of knowledge and the awareness of health professionals, as well as those who contribute to shaping social stances and mentalities regarding the defining importance of the early human experiences.

In conclusion, may I go back to the starting point of this text: A civilized society should be able to ponder, plan and adopt measures for the future citizens not only after they will have fallen ill but at the dawn of their psychic life, in other words during the pregnancy at the latest.

References

Bennett H.A., Einarson A., Taddio A., Koren G., Einarson T.R. (2004) Prevalence of Depression During Pregnancy: Systematic Review. *Obstetrics & Gynecology* 103: 698–709.

Bauer A., Parsonage M., Knapp M., Iemmi V., Adelaja B. (2014) *The Costs of Perinatal Mental Health Problems*. London: Centre for Mental Health and London School of Economics.

Bydlowski M. (1991) La transparence psychique de la grossesse. *Etudes Freudiennes* 32: 135–142.

Faisal-Cury A., Rossi Menezes P. (2007) Prevalence of Anxiety and Depression during Pregnancy in a Private Setting Sample. *Arch. Womens Ment. Health. 10*: 25–32.

Karmaliani R., Asad N., Bann C.M., *et al.* (2009) Prevalence of Anxiety, Depression and Associated Factors among Pregnant Women of Hyderabad, Pakistan. *The International Journal of Social Psychiatry* 55(5). doi:10.1177/0020764008094645.

Mayes L. (2005) Parental Attachment Systems: Neural Circuits, Genes and Experiential Contributions to Parental Engagement. *Clinical Neuroscience Research*, 4: 301–313.

Meltzer-Brody S. (2011) New Insights into Perinatal Depression: Pathogenesis and Treatment during Pregnancy and Postpartum. *Dialogues Clin. Neuros.* 13(1): 89–100.

Parsons C.E., Young K.S., Rochat T.J., Kringelbach M.L., Stein A. (2012) Postnatal Depression and its Effects on Child Development: A Review of Evidence from Low- and Middle-Income Countries. *British Medical Bulletin*, 101(1): 57.

Raphael-Leff J. (1993) *Pregnancy: The Inside Story*. London: Karnac.

Salomonson B. (2018) *Psychodynamic Interventions in Pregnancy and Infancy: Clinical and Theoretical Perspectives*. London: Routledge.

Teixeira C., Figueiredo B., Conde A., Pacheco A., Costa R. (2009) Anxiety and Depression during Pregnancy in Women and Men. *J. Affect. Disord.* 119: 142–148.

Chapter 4

Cruel Fate

Jennifer Davids

> Nevertheless, the majority of child patients in the hospital, whether acutely or chronically ill, will benefit greatly from any plan under which the needs of their minds are considered to be as important as the needs of their bodies.
> (Anna Freud in Bergman and Freud, 1965, p. 151)

> Those of us who have the luck to enjoy good health forget about this vast parallel universe of the unwell – their daily miseries, their banal ordeals. Only when you cross that frontier into the world of ill-health do you recognize its quiet, massive presence, its breeding permanence.
> (Boyd, 2009, p. 415)

> The smell and sounds of the paediatric ward where I worked 30 years ago come back to me. Smells of sweat, disinfectant, other unpleasant pungent odours difficult to characterise, the smell of uneaten food wheeled away in the trolleys. Sounds of hasty feet on the linoleum floors responding to calls, of curtains speedily drawn round beds, of quiet serious voices, machine beeps, family arguments, the flurry of doctors' ward rounds, and sometimes the loudest sound of all, silence.
> (Davids, 2020)

Introduction

For many years some child psychoanalysts and psychotherapists have offered helpful, thoughtful interventions to physically ill children and adolescents as both in- and out-patients. Anna Freud collaborated with paediatricians and collaborated on a classic book *Children in Hospital* with Bergman. Winnicott too worked with sick, hospitalised children as a paediatrician and later as a child and adult psychoanalyst. Both Anna Freud and Winnicott believed in the importance of the emotional welfare of physically ill children. When stressed and overwhelmed by the realities of serious illness, children can regress and lose their ability to cope. In such times of crisis they may well benefit from "mental first-aid" (Bergman in Bergman and Freud, 1965). It is at such moments of lowered defence that the clinician can reach the perplexed and often isolated child to contain some of his thoughts, feelings, conflicts, primitive terrors and anguish, as well as provide understanding of his unconscious dilemmas. Such moments can be "moments of meeting" (Stern, 2004) which go some way to transforming the child's lonely anguish making it more sensible and bearable. I argue that the clinician needs to be adaptable with respect to her setting, able to hold on to her internal setting and analytic identity, as well as use a flexible technique. The ill child needs to be met on a level which he, at that moment, can tolerate, and where his most pressing needs can be named and understood. By coming to understand and accept his bodily states as well as his mental states, he has more on his side to weather the storms of his illness and the treatment. Being helped to acknowledge the truths of this testing journey together with developing and holding onto realistic hopes, frees the ill child. The literature on the subject is expanding worldwide with work in the USA, (Bluebond-Langner, 1978; Furman, 1984; Katz, 2020; Kliman, 1968), in the UK (Pauline Cohen, 1990; Margaret Cohen, 2003; Emmanuel et al., 1990; Elfer and Lee, 2009; Hinton, 1980; Judd, 1989; Moran, 1984) and in South Africa (Frenkel, 2004) to name a few. Such work is demanding but immensely rewarding.

My Initial Interest

Before I began my training in psychoanalysis, Enid Balint knowing of my interest in primitive states of the mind, suggested that I might consider working in a hospital with ill patients where I might see and understand states of regression. I bore this in mind when some years later after qualifying, I applied to work as a child and adolescent psychotherapist in paediatrics. There I learnt much about primitive states of the body and mind and the essential link between soma and psyche. I also learnt about primitive and social defences (Menzies Lyth, 1970) on the part of patients, their families and medical staff on the ward.

The Ward – a New World and Finding a Place

My first days and weeks as a new kid on the block were spent getting to know the lay of the land rather like an anthropologist learning about a new culture or an immigrant arriving in a new country. I too had to learn a new language of medical terms and abbreviations as well as noting the militaristic style of the language medical staff frequently used in the war against the diseases, such as when an increased dosage or change of medication "should zap it". This work setting felt very different to me – a huge hospital like a city with a life of its own. It felt rather like a railway station with passengers trying to locate their train – in this context their ward, clinic, their doctors. It felt different from when I worked in the psychiatric department of a general hospital or in a hospital devoted to the treatment of mental illness. It took me some months to find my place, perhaps a journey sharing some similarities to those experienced by child patients and their families.

The skills I had learned in infant, toddler and nursery school observation stood me in good stead as I watched and learnt about this new world where I had chosen to land. I saw some of the non-verbal communication that went on (e.g. the quick looks passing between parents and children, between doctors, and between children, which often followed difficult to take in news, and conveyed more than a thousand words). The atmosphere on the ward was palpable and a helpful barometer of the anxieties carried by patients and staff. I had not realised how many severely ill children there would be on the ward. I was called "a Psych" and initially some children and families questioned whether I had any use. I felt marginalised rather like the uncomfortable thoughts and feelings they would have liked to push to one side. And there were times overtaken by a sense of helplessness, when I found myself wishing that I was a doctor who could *do* something. I realised how I had lost the child and become disease-led rather than child-led, again mirroring the parents' and children's responses. In time I recovered my belief in my role as providing a space where emotional experience and mental pain could be listened to, digested and understood. Margaret Cohen (2003), a child psychotherapist working on a neonatal intensive care unit (NICU), argues that medical people in a work situation like the NICU have to "emphasize the practical, the rational, the real, the sane, in order to get on with their work, while the psychotherapist will be more aware of the non-rational, the imaginative, fantasy and the insane" (p. 10).

I hopefully played some part in helping some of the child patients and families weather and process the storms they were going through. In this chapter I will focus on two such children and not discuss my work with other less critically ill children.

I quickly realised that I was not welcome on the ward; this inhospitality came particularly from the nursing staff who regarded me with suspicion, a fly by night who worked on the ward only part-time. The busy consultants who came and went from the ward, were in the main more welcoming, less threatened by my presence and my psychological knowledge. The hospital school staff were friendlier colleagues from whom I learnt much; they had often known the patients and their families through many relapses and past stays on the ward. They represented a kind of continuity, links to ordinary educational life and to the children's schools.

The nursing staff however seemed to doubt that I would stay the course. I often felt like an unnecessary outsider. The nurses seemed to belong to an exclusive club from which I was walled off; a kind of siege mentality keeping me out. I realised as time went on that this defensiveness was their way of protecting themselves. Many of them were young and in the staff group which I came to run, I heard often about their having lost young relatives to cancer themselves. Interestingly the junior doctors, as they came to recognise my ongoing presence, used to spontaneously talk very briefly and intensely to me in the elevator going up to the ward. They revealed their tremendous anxieties and distress in these brief intense conversations but immediately the doors opened on to the level of the ward, they raised their professional personas, masking all their feelings in front of the other medical staff. I recall one particular ward round led by a very experienced oncologist. I noticed as we sat in a circle that one of the young doctors had borrowed the hamster from the hospital school room and was stroking it, as we listened to the grave reviews of the very ill patients. I thought the doctor was seeking comfort to hold himself together against his own shock and helplessness. There was often a manic atmosphere on the ward with the staff joking and flirting. I came to understand this as their way of hanging onto life especially when there were many re-admissions and news of deaths. Christmas was a particularly difficult time for the families and the staff. Again I noticed how the young medical staff who had formed strong attachments to some patients, bought expensive gifts for them. These gifts were usually medium-size cuddly toys. I wondered whether these were rather desperate attempts to compensate and comfort themselves, literally with something soft, for the guilt about sometimes having to physically hurt their patients (and about not being able to help their patients more). The medical staff also seemed identified with the children's miserable states of mind and body, and cutting disappointment about having to spend a national holiday in the hospital. The loss of ordinariness and normal life was a recurrent theme.

As I became a presence on the ward, it was agreed that a small room, which had been a bathroom, would be cleared for me to see patients and parents. It had a sliding door with a lock and the walls were painted yellow. I remember calling it "The Yellow Submarine", a name which the children adopted. An interesting choice of a name of a Beatles song for children. I wonder whether it reflected my sense of being enclosed in a small space, in the world of illness and trauma, as well as being under the surface, in touch with the unconscious. From a submerged submarine one can view the surface; submarines can emerge from the depths, rather like lurking unconscious thoughts and feelings coming into awareness by being put into words. Sometimes I would arrive to find the space filled with boxes of medical supplies, reflecting the staff's ambivalence, if not hostility, towards my presence. Much of the time when the children were confined to their beds or bays, I had to create my own setting by drawing the curtains around their bed. I had to be flexible often putting up with interruptions by medical staff needing to carry out necessary interventions. I learnt to hold onto my own internal setting. The most important thing was my emotional contact with the patients and their families. It was a quite a learning curve, and mirrored to some degree the huge adaptation the child patients and families had to make as well as the learning curves forced on them by cruel fate.

There were a range of experiences that I was faced with. Firstly the severity of the diagnoses and the knowledge that cancer cells can multiply and spread very fast in children. The sense of interruption of these children's lives and the feeling that something was out of joint were powerful. I felt that some natural order of things had been reversed; inwardly I protested: "It's not fair! They are far too young to be so ill and even die". I realised the series of uncertainties they faced, together with the sense of waiting and boredom. The children seemed and were isolated, sometimes looking blank and spaced out, marooned in their worlds. Some have described talking to the ceiling or indeed themselves in such situations. In addition they faced the complicated dilemma of being dependent on medical staff who sometimes had to hurt them in order to help them. Often their anger had to be hidden as they needed the painful investigations and treatment. So much had to be endured. At times it seemed that they were being tested to their very limits. And I had to learn how to witness this sometimes or be open to enter, share and hear about their experiences, acknowledging their mental pain and fear. I also learned to respect their defences, as well as those of their parents.

At the time I worked in other settings including a child analytic clinic, a university college and in private practice. This provided something of a balance although sometimes the transition on the same day back to working with physically healthier children was difficult in that I noticed that I felt how unfair life was. I was filled with and carrying powerful emotions stirred up on the ward. I realised that I was experiencing much of what the hospitalised children did namely anger, helplessness, loss and sadness about how different their lives had become. On very bad days I was aware of thoughts like, "What have these kids got to complain about – they are physically well" and had to pull myself back to remain conscious of their mental pain. It was helpful when staff in the common room who had worked in hospital settings and who were interested in my paediatric work, asked how things were going, probably sensing my dilemmas.

My reactions were not only confined to work; sometimes I noticed a spill-over at home. My husband commented on the numerous bottles of fresh orange juice I was buying and my need to purchase so many vegetables and super foods. I realised that I was frightened of our getting ill and was concretely trying to ward off vulnerability by trying to build our immunity. Sometimes he sensed my sadness, perplexity and rage and sensitively suggested listening to Mahler, Beethoven and my favourite, Rachmaninov. Another resource were the phone calls from my mother who inquired how the work at the hospital was going; she had nursed her own mother who had suffered from and died of cancer in her early fifties. My father kept more of a distance, but sometimes asked how my poetry was going, when did I last go to the theatre, and gently but firmly reminded me of my need to maintain a work-life balance. I was fortunate that the people closest to me, although somewhat concerned about the toll the work was taking on me, knew me well, acted as resources as well as pointing me to sources of replenishment; I knew they deeply respected my work. It is interesting that it has taken me so many long years to write rather than talk and present this work, something similar to Katz (2020) who discusses the multiple meanings of her need to write a paper many years after her work with a dying child had passed.

Case 1: Sebastian

I have called this boy Sebastian as his family reminded me of the character of Sebastian and his Catholic family in Evelyn Waugh's *Brideshead Revisited*. Similar to that fictional family the theme of guilt was prevalent in this patient's family.

Sebastian's grandmother latched onto me during my early days on the ward. She quickly established that I was neither a parent or relative, nor a member of the medical team. I don't think she really took in that I was "a Psych", as she called me. She used me to evacuate into. The fact that I was young and could have been her daughter was a factor too. She seemed very lonely and slightly dishevelled in her dress and appearance. Her greying, often unkempt, hair was striking. She spent much time on the ward with her grandson, confiding in me that her son and daughter were such busy people with a large family so she was happy to be there and anyway she was, "very close to Sebastian". Interestingly I hardly ever saw evidence of this intimacy. Sebastian was strikingly withdrawn, in his own world, often caught up with watching television, socialising with his brothers and sometimes the other patients and staff on the ward. He was clearly no stranger to the staff, an experienced child patient who had been hospitalised on the same ward several times before. He was in after another relapse. Diagnosis: leukaemia.

Granny told me that her husband had died about a year before so she was on her own. She said, "It should be me in that bed, not him ... It's the wrong way around." Other times she confided how she was preparing for her own death, saying she no longer needed new clothes, she had sufficient to last her remaining days. She intimated that her son's marriage was not a happy one despite all their material success and wealth. "I don't know what we have done to deserve this ... poor Sebastian, he's done nothing wrong." It was clear she believed that Sebastian's cancer was a punishment for some wrong doings in and by the family. Her sense of being haunted by death was palpable as was her depression which she tried to conceal. She saw my wedding ring and wanted to know whether I had children and then quickly apologised for being "nosey"; "I get the feeling", she told me, "that you'd be a committed, good mother and not put your career first like some people seem to do".

Sebastian kept himself largely to himself; he struck me as small almost wizened. I knew he was 9 years old, but he looked pale, tense and shrunken. He was very watchful of the goings-on around him. I sometimes sensed an anger in him. He kept his distance from me and seemed in a bubble of his family and the social circle of hospital mates and staff.

I knew that Sebastian and other children on the ward used the Yellow Submarine, to talk at night and over the weekends when I was not there. They told me that they talked about "private stuff ... You know what's going to happen ... the doctors ... football ... heaven and hell". Interestingly Bluebond-Langer describes how children used the bathroom on the ward to share similar concerns.

One time Sebastian was reported to be very low. He had crawled under his bed and would not come out, saying he just wanted to die. The staff and family were desperate. They could not identify any triggers to his current state of mind. The consultant paediatrician asked me if I could try to help.

Vignette I

I drew curtains around his bed.

JD: S, it's JD. I know you're under your bed and don't really want to speak to anyone.

I heard him kick or punch the underside of the bed.

S: Go away.

I heard him crying which I found very painful to hear.

JD: Those sound like very lonely, frightened tears.

Silence

JD: Can I come sit next to you on the floor?
S: Don't care what you do. You can't do anything anyway.
JD: Okay, I am going to sit on the floor.

I do, I look under his bed and fleetingly make eye contact with him. He is curled up in a foetus-like position.

S: It's probably dirty.

Silence

S: I am never going to get better.
JD: That's an awful feeling.

Silence

S: I am going to burn.
JD: Burn?
S: Yip ... in Hell that's what happens when you die. You burn in Hell.
JD: What makes you think you are going to Hell?

Pause. More crying and hitting.

S: Because I am bad. Bad people go to Hell, that's it. That is what happens.
JD: In what way do you feel you are bad?

Silence

S: Things I did. I didn't do my homework. I stole from my friend. I wished my parents dead. If it wasn't for me, they would probably be happier. They are sick of this cancer and this hospital ... I know they are.
JD: I think you certainly are sick of being sick and in this hospital.
S: Am

More kicking.

S: I just want to die ... I am not going to eat ... I am not taking any more medicine ... nothing.
JD: Sounds like you are sick of fighting and feel that there is nothing much you can do or anyone can do, so you blame yourself ... and think the cancer is all your fault and a kind of punishment.
S: Maybe.

Long Silence of several minutes.

S: Your socks have got green in them.
JD: Hm.
S: You like colours ... green and yellow ... like the Yellow Submarine.
JD: True.
S: It must be uncomfortable sitting on the floor ...
JD: I don't mind.

Silence

S: It's not so comfortable under here. Maybe I can watch *The A-Team*? Will you watch with me?
JD: For a while.
S: Close your eyes and count until I say Stop.

I do what he has asked.

S: Stop!

I realise he's on his bed and looking for the TV remote control.

We find the channel and watch for a little while. I say I am going to leave him now. He seems engrossed in the programme but waves goodbye.

Here we see how Sebastian already feels he is in hell: his tortured state and ongoing self-torment, along with his anguish, terror and despair, are palpable. He tries to regain some control by refusing to speak and move – this is a theme Emmanuel et al. (1990) have identified as common in the experienced of children facing life-threatening illness. The illness is experienced as invasive, stealing a child's agency, his freedom and ultimately even his life. Sebastian's punitive persecutory superego is manifest; perhaps an identification with the belief system of his grandmother and family. He seems to harbour a belief that *you only get better if you have behaved well, been a good boy and have never put a foot wrong*. Sebastian seemed to equate being ill with being bad. I think part of his wish to hide was motivated by his profound sense of shame. My technique included my naming and containing his almost unbearable feelings, a literal coming down to his level on the floor, and symbolically, to his state of mind and body. Sebastian was in a dark place, a state of breakdown. There was something confessional in his words as if he was treating me as a priest, unconsciously asking for absolution. However, he takes in what I say and seems to be able to recover his interest in the Other, noticing the colour in my socks and referring to my room, a kind of container and a place where people meet and talk about "private stuff". Sebastian seems to come alive, starts to re-engage, re-finding the colour in the listening, receiving Other, through this brief intervention of my feeling with him and verbalising some of his affective states. I was trying to metabolise some of his raw experiences, rather like a mother digesting and representing her infant's pain. Perhaps the interpretation of his rage and disappointment along with his attempt to blame himself brought some relief and literally helped him come out from under. He was able to re-emerge onto his hospital bed and resume the fight, turning to his usual defences of escape into fantasy via watching television. *The A-Team* was a television series about soldiers of fortune who fight bravely, often against the odds. I have found that this coping mechanism of identifying with male heroes is quite common in hospitalised young boys who feel castrated and emasculated by their illness. The burning is interesting; I wondered whether it was linked in his mind to times when he suffered from very high temperatures, as is common in childhood leukaemia, and literally felt that he was burning up.

However, as Sebastian's condition worsened the doctors began to talk about the need for a bone marrow transplant and a donor. It was at this point that he indicated that he wanted to talk to me. Granny had told me that he was more withdrawn than usual, that something seemed to be on his mind and asked again for my help.

Vignette 2

JD: Hello. You want to talk to me, I hear.
S: Yeah. I am not mad, okay.
JD: Okay.
S: Well, you know I am going to have a bone marrow transplant. And my brother has been tested and they found out that he can be a donor. He says he does not mind, so I guess that's cool. Although it will hurt when they take it out of him. But he knows.

Silence.

S: Well, I have been thinking ... maybe this sounds weird ... Will I no longer like lamb chops? It's my favourite food.
JD: You seem to be wondering whether you are going to change somehow.
S: Yeah ... the thing is he likes pizza and baked beans and I don't ... can't stand the stuff ... But if his stuff is inside me ... will I starting liking what he does? [S looks upset]
JD: I think you are telling me that you are worried that you are going to lose your identity, being you, and that you'll become your brother and you don't want that.
S: Yip.
JD: I don't think that will actually happen, but you might want to talk about it to the doctors.
S: They'll laugh at me.
JD: You are afraid they won't understand.
S: Yes.

I heard the next day that Sebastian had already asked the doctors concerned. They had responded in a sensitive way, reassuring him that this was not the case. He had apparently laughed, saying that he would still support a different football team from his brother then!

Sebastian was worried about losing control, being thought mad. Here we can see how trying to understand his bodily state profoundly impacts on his mental state. His guilt about his brother having to be hurt is conscious; perhaps his unconscious guilt about taking or stealing from his brother is less available to him. Sebastian wonders whether this new substance will wipe out his core sense of self, that he will lose being the Sebastian he knows himself to be. Castelnuovo-Tedesco (1973) in an interesting paper describes how an organ transplant *adds* something. He argues that the self unconsciously experiences the new acquisition as an introject, as an object or part-object that immediately becomes affectively active. During regressed mental states, guilt about having "stolen" the organ may occur together with the feeling that essential characteristics have been altered as a result of possessing, inside, a part from another human being.

Sebastian feared that he would lose his identity, his sense of self. He concretely feared that he would be taken over by his brother's marrow, become him and no longer feel himself to be in his own bones made of his own stuff, his likes and dislikes. Already in a state of regression during a relapse, such terrors and preoccupations were more apparent. We can see his states of mind and body. I helped Sebastian to face the reality of his situation proportionately. I listened to his fantasies taking them seriously, interpreted some deeper fears about losing his self-object differentiation and his fears of merging. I also helped him to differentiate fantasy from reality. I suggested he talk to the doctors to get the needed information and do a reality check. Through this work Sebastian was able to integrate the addition of his brother's donation; he had to find a *psychological fit* by knowing that he would not lose aspects of his character.

My interventions facilitated the restoration of his coping and returning him to the primary care of the medical staff particularly the nursing staff. Faced with his regression, despair and angry refusal, the nursing staff felt helpless and withdrew from him. I needed to help them re-discover their empathy for him which they had temporarily lost under fire. They could then resume their roles as care takers of the patient. Sebastian had his transplant and was isolated on the ward which he knew well. I believe that he had a successful outcome.

Case 2: Akin

I have named the second boy I am going to discuss "Akin", which is the Yoruban name meaning heroic or brave. From very early on in my acquaintance with him, Akin brought to my mind an image of a strong young African warrior standing on a rock holding up his spear, ready for battle. Akin shared a dignity and pride with this masculine figure in my mind. I soon became aware of his quiet presence and his fighting spirit. I recall seeing his mother also strikingly proud, sitting next to his bed and the quiet communication between them. They seemed to share a deep, painful understanding. To this day I admire their dignity and the courageous ways they attempted to face Akin's grave illness.

I learnt that 10-year-old Akin had been recently admitted, that he was diagnosed with lymphoblastic leukaemia and that he was finishing a course of chemotherapy. He greeted me when I first passed by his bay, and said hello. His mother greeted me too. They regarded me with slight anxiety – was I another doctor? Another one to deal with? I explained that I was a child psychotherapist. Mother raised an eyebrow. She recognised my accent, saying, "You're not British. Where do you come from?" Akin said, "Australia?" I answered, "No." Mother then ventured, "New Zealand?" I said, "No." And then they both said at the same time "South Africa." So through this guessing game they placed me. I said, "African like you." They smiled. I asked where they came from. "Nigeria." I sensed somehow that they felt a long way from home. We were connected by our African identity and feeling a long way from our origins. We were also both new to the ward and to "the parallel universe" (Boyd, 2009) of childhood cancer.

Mother spontaneously chatted to me during the next few weeks. She told me she had a scientific background and that her ex-husband, Akin's father was living in Africa. She looked sad and I sensed her loneliness. With some excitement the doctors discharged Akin and they left the hospital with mother looking relieved and Akin so happy to be going home to "good food", looking forward to seeing his friends again and even the stimulation of school. Apparently he was a diligent student with high ambitions. Some months later I noticed that they were back. Mother's ironic comment, "Here we are again", revealed her concern and disappointment. There followed a period of waiting for test results and then the confirmation that the leukaemia was back. I saw her shock and her holding back her tears, after the doctors spoke to her. During the next few days she kept the doctors at a distance clearly angry with them. She looked sullen, unlike her usual calm demeanour. I noticed myself feeling helpless and angry too. I saw her toughening herself up, bracing herself for what lay ahead for her beloved son.

Akin, looked vulnerable, worried and sometimes I observed irritable exchanges between the two of them, arguing about his leaving his food uneaten. Even food Mother had brought from home. He said, "I am not hungry. I don't want it … I can't eat it." I could see the hurt expression in her eyes. One day Akin waved to me as I walked by. I realised I could not stand next to his bed. He was surrounded by his laminar flow the purpose of which he explained to me. He looked bored, confined to his space and again enduring an unwelcome situation. He told me he was bored and I responded that I could understand that and that I guessed he might feel a bit imprisoned having to stay in his marked out area. He gave me a small smile.

The next time I saw him I saw fear in his eyes: he was shivering and looked very unwell. The nurses were running around trying to find him more blankets. They kept on taking his temperature and I heard a word I did not know – neutropenic. Akin's teeth were literally chattering as he held himself together under the numerous blankets. He looked as if he felt he was freezing to death. Hours later I learnt that he was febrile, burning with a very high temperature. I could see that he sensed the staff's anxiety. I sensed how he felt terrified, trapped in his sick changeable body.

The following day things seemed a little calmer – the haematologists had been in. Mother was very quiet. She looked exhausted and had slept next to

Akin's bed the previous night. Akin was sleeping. She said she was going to the hospital chapel downstairs and asked, "Will you come with me?" We went down together. She lit a candle and I followed suit, following her lead. We sat in silence. I remember the semi-darkness of the chapel and the sense of stillness and peace. I presumed she was praying. We did not exchange a word; I said after some time that I would leave her there as I needed to go. She nodded and mouthed thank you.

The next two or three weeks were erratic. Akin confided to me how bored he felt and I sometimes caught a glimpse of the healthy boy he once was – his quickness of mind, his wish to run, jump and dream carefreely, his mischievousness and his warm sense of humour. One day he showed me the board game he and the night nurse had constructed together. I teased him saying, "So you have found another way of being bored." He laughed gently.

The board game communicates so much of Akin's world, external and internal, his understanding of these worlds and his responses to them.

With this board game this latency boy showed his detailed observations and knowledge as well as his attempt to master the experiences of his illness and of being hospitalised. It was his attempt to organise his experiences in a meaningful structure, to map it and show the setbacks and progressions in his journey with his illness while in hospital.

The game drawn on two joined pieces of cardboard consists of a number of squares. There are accompanying cards of Doctors' Visits and Menu Cards (see Figure 4.1). Players (and interestingly there were four coloured counters) move around according to the roll of the dice like so many board games. Yet the roll of the dice captures the sense of unpredictability of where one lands – what I call Cruel Fate. Progress is not straightforward: there are backward and forward moves – progressions and disappointing setbacks in this new life which requires so much adaptation. There are opportunities for a lucky break and equally cards which bring bad news. Some examples of doctor's visits are cell count and going to theatre while Menu cards include take-ins from McDonalds and food from home. Looked at from afar one realises that the shape of the board game is an injection needle or syringe. It also looks like a rocket and the final destination is HOME. The drawing conveys Akin's deep longing for discharge and a return home. On the left top corner are drawn three bottles, two of which show their labels – Mouth Wash and Blood.

The Game begins with Start – Admitted into Hospital. On either side at the bottom is the ambulance and the welcoming nurse. Interestingly the nurse stands in a way that reminds me of a muscular Popeye. There is also a drawing of an ambulance with its siren. The first square is about the bed and then subsequent squares about which bay one will be assigned to. The squares reveal the ups and downs of illness and hospital life particularly its unpredictability. Doctor visits are linked to a set of cards outlining various possibilities over which there is little control (e.g. neutrophils up so

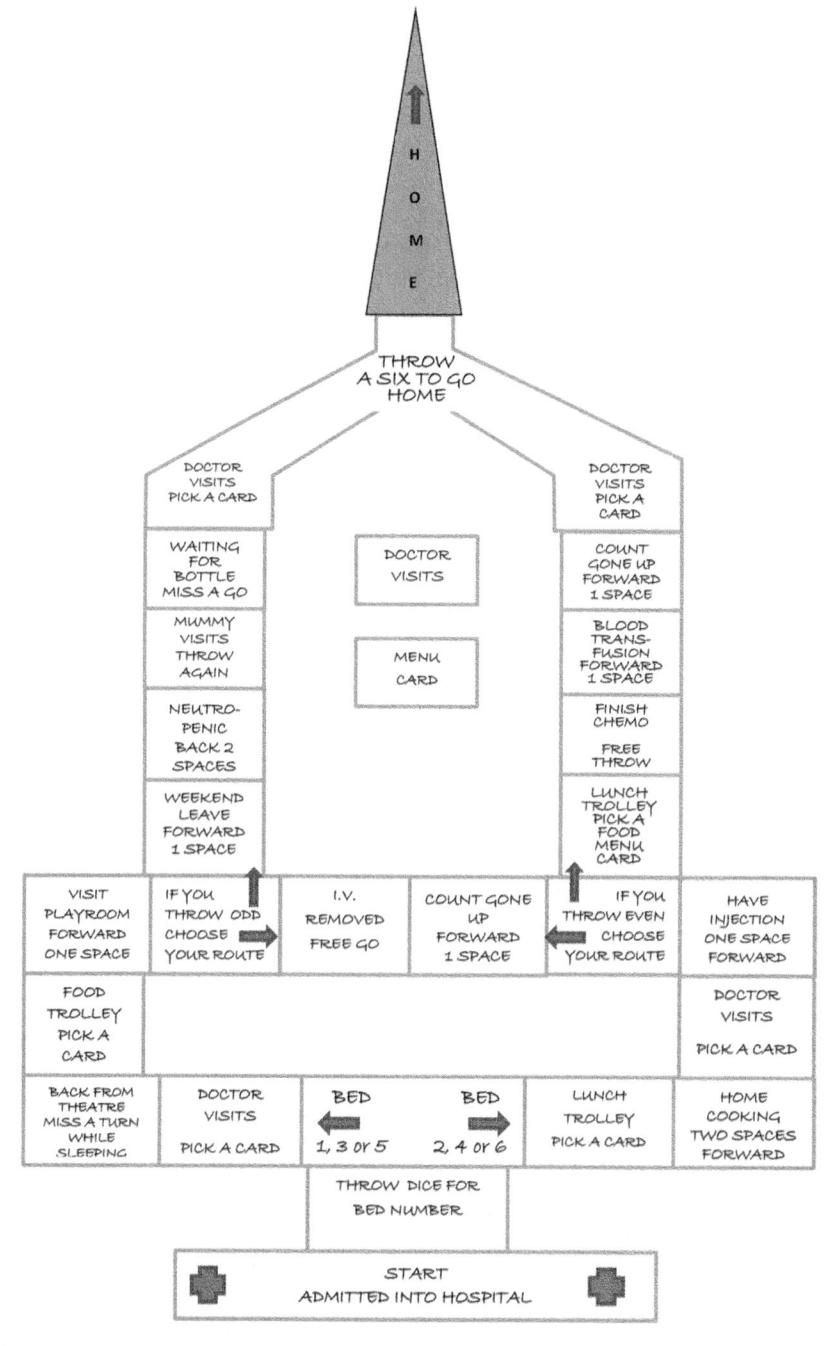

Figure 4.1 Diagram based on Akin's board game
Source: Jennifer Davids, 2021

permission to leave laminar flow, canula being fitted, going to theatre, declared well and discharge). A second set of cards are Menu cards which show us how important food becomes to the child patient. This set shows us how the patient still has some choice. It also shows us disgust with some food. Food seems to represent choice, life and some kind of precious normality. The squares include waiting for bottle, blood transfusion, visits to playroom, weekend leave, injections. The game also contains throws of the dice which can lead to progress. This seems to be Akin's wishful way of trying to find ways of mastering and magically controlling his journey. The game constructed with the help of a male night nurse shows us Akin's creativity and his communication of what it like to have to play this life game. A game that was not a game. Furman (1984) writes about the sophisticated and creative activities dying children seek out and enjoy when they feel their sense of dying is shared and that their comfort is shared.

Painting pictures, composing songs, and building models are all ways of expressing their experience and may be mementoes for the future, proofs that even a short life is worth living and can fulfil some promise. In my experience this pertains to children struggling to come to terms with life-threatening illness.

Later it became clear what the next step was going to be in Akin's treatment – bone marrow transplant. But at a different hospital. Before he left, Akin said he wanted me to have this board game. I felt very moved and honoured. I thought Akin's gift of his game was his way of communicating his experiences to me. He knew that I knew that it was not just a game. I also think he knew I would treasure it and help him to communicate it as a kind of legacy, of leaving his mark on the world. Akin's gift at a point of separation, was his way of saying "Keep this. Remember me."

His mother subsequently contacted me to ask me to visit him at this hospital. I remember both journeys, the outward filled with anticipation, and the return. It was a big modern cottage style hospital and eventually I found the right building and his room at the end of a very silent corridor, in isolation. The door had a glass porthole and staff had to follow strict hygiene procedures as well as wear gowns, masks and gloves to enter so as to reduce the risk of infection. He seemed to be in a protective womb, facilitating a new life, resembling a re-birth, with this new bone marrow. I gestured through the glass window asking him if he wanted me to come in and he indicated not. I waited while he was examined. And then we communicated through the porthole window by pen and cardboard, the same materials as the board game. Clearly pleased to see me, and hungry for stimulation in his isolation, he wanted to know how I got to the hospital, did it take long to get there, etc. His mother looked thinner, exhausted, tense and thanked me so much for coming. Akin wrote, "I am OK". I remember struggling with wanting to hold this boy. Again I was struck by Akin's bravery and wish to live. On the way home I cried and inwardly wished him strength and recovery.

Sometime later I heard that he did not make it. I felt immensely sad. I found and looked again at his gift, the board game. It was a goodbye gift, at the time of leaving the ward he had come to know so well. Akin also wanted to make sure that I would remember him by giving me the game. I think he knew that I took in his experience and knew much of what he was going through. He knew that I knew. Was it also a kind of legacy? In retrospect when I heard of his death, I wondered whether Akin knew at some level that he might be going home, going to his final resting place, back to his origins so to speak. Again the image of the proud African warrior came to me.

Houlding (2018) describes her reflections on the sudden loss of a female analytic patient who developed cancer and died. Norton (1963) movingly writes about an adult patient's gift of a red dress to her which she understood as symbolising life and sexuality. I think part of my writing this chapter is my way of mourning my young patient and sharing the gift of his communication of some of his experiences of being treated for his leukaemia.

Discussion

In this chapter I have described aspects of my journey towards finding my role and place on a general paediatric ward. The atmosphere on the ward seemed to be affected by rapid staff-turnover, the personalities of senior nursing staff and the number of seriously ill and dying children. Modern medicine has advanced making bone marrow transplants much better and more successful procedures than before. More child-friendly and parent-friendly procedures in bone marrow transplants have developed, for example, dedicated rooms with negative air pressure so that the outside possibly contaminated air is pushed out on entry enable parents to take turns to stay with their isolated children. Professionals including child psychotherapists now assess the "best interests" of donors and the procedure both for donor and recipient is carefully explained (Elfer, personal communication, 2020).

I have also tried to show how two boys aged 9 and 10 did much thinking as they responded to their Cruel Fate and to living in a world apart, this parallel world of illness as described by Boyd (2009). Enid Balint was right in pointing out that I would learn much about regressed states of mind in working with ill patients in the hospital setting. I also learnt much about regressed states of the body when these two boys felt stripped to the core, deprived of their autonomy, exposed to extreme situations by their illnesses and their treatments. Sometimes I felt like a helpless mother witnessing her child's pain and fear as when Akin's temperature plummeted and then soared, making him feel he was freezing or frying to death. Sebastian too conveyed his terror and his literally being laid low by his illness and by his fantasies about punishment and the after-life. In order to help these children, their families and the staff, I had to do much work within myself. This inner work included facing my responses to life-threatening illness, to helplessness and to early death. I had to accept my own survivor guilt, my different Fate. This work was essential to help me listen to their pain, to tune into their unconscious communications, to follow their lead and help them maintain realistic hope. These were some of the constituents of these moments of meeting at times of crisis. Cohen (1990) describes the aim of simple timely interventions by child psychotherapists in hospital work as *restoring the capacity of the child patient to cope* through containing and making meaning of unremitting regressive or self-destructive behaviour which can interfere with the medical treatment and the healing process. Katz (2020) argues that the therapist of a dying child can function as an "other" who can help in working "to recognise or acknowledge distressing, unintegrated or unspeakable internal states and self-representations" (p. 165). I agree that this pertains to working with children with life-threatening illnesses. I argue that the child psychotherapist needs to be something of an outsider, who can bear what might be seen as irrational even insane by the medical team, who are more focused on the pragmatic and rational aspects of the treatment. They need such defences to do their difficult jobs. The staff felt Sebastian was untreatable when he withdrew and refused their help. As described, my task was to bring my skills to help him with his extreme states of mind and mental pain. I then talked with the nurses helping them to understand his "irrational" behaviour and his plight; they could then recover their empathy and resume their caretaking roles.

I take my hat off to both Sebastian and Akin. They both developed admirable coping skills. I saw them at times when their coping was threatened if not broken down. Not coping and feeling out of control affect self-esteem. Their bodies had let them down so badly and they felt unprotected by their parents who could not stop or shield them from the illness and its sequelae. Their self and body representations underwent change affecting their self-esteem, making them feel different, damaged and even worthless. Katz (2020) highlights how the ability to understand oneself and the other can be compromised by the disorganising impact of terminal illness. She describes how these changing self- representations affect both the physical self in the face of a weakening body, and the sense of self-agency in the face of loss of control to illness and medical staff who intrude on the patient's autonomy.

Close relationships can be altered in the face of serious illness, painful investigations and treatments. Under such threat the need for physical and emotional comfort may be heightened. Preoccupied parents may not be able to respond to such needs. So the child may feel isolated, lonely, overwhelmed and even panicked. Regressed states of mind and body have to be faced and contained, and here I believe is one area where psychoanalytically trained child psychotherapists can play a vital role. Sometimes interventions can be made on a verbal level, helping to make some meaning of the child's experience. The psychotherapist on the ward may also have to bear very powerful projections which may be communicated on a non-verbal level. Some of my work with parents for example accompanying Akin's mother to the hospital chapel was on a non-verbal level yet constituted a deep level of communication. Much of the work of the child psychotherapist is helping the patient and family bear the near unbearable and the uncertain.

Both young boys sometimes grappled with understanding their predicament: "I am very ill. Why?" They were faced with existential questions. Goldie and Desmarais (2005) and Straker (2013) have described this dilemma in work with ill and dying adult patients. These two boys both came from religious families – Sebastian seemed to have identified with the beliefs of his Granny, tormented by a persecutory sense of Catholic guilt, whilst Akin's mother turned in her own individual way to her beliefs which seemed to offer some solace. I felt that both Sebastian's granny and Akin's mother turned to me as a kind of partner with whom to share their experiences and to help them reach their children. Sebastian was a seasoned patient, battle-weary and traumatised. He seemed more hardened to his experiences. In states of regression, Sebastian communicated his helplessness and hopelessness, despairing that no one could help him. He also revealed his thinking about why he had leukaemia. He believed he was being punished for being bad. Akin was at a different stage, newer to the experiences of being so ill. He was more open and more object-related. For the most part he was able to contain himself and use his defences to help himself actively face some of the traumatic aspects of his illness. Both boys seemed to be battling to hold on to precious aspects of their own selves, to not be taken over by the leukaemia which they perceived as a foreign body invading and destroying them. They used both active and passive defences, sometimes dissociating, freezing (Fraiberg, 1982) and blanking out. Often a distinction is drawn between fate and destiny. Destiny is seen as the way one actively responds to one's fate. Bollas (1989) has written about the destiny drive.

Both boys lost much of normal life. For long periods they lived in a hospital not at home or school. Their lives were interrupted and could at worst be cut short. In such a situation children have to mourn the possible loss of the future (i.e. their dreams, desires and aspirations). At times I sensed their envy of my health and future and also that I had had a childhood imagined to be a normal one. I too had to face the unpredictable odds and unfair Cruel Fate, for example, how Sebastian was helped by his transplant whereas Akin did not make it through. For the first time in my clinical practice I had to face the death of a child patient. I had to think and reflect very deeply about my own limits, the prospect of my own death, as well as acknowledge how much life can be lived fully even in the most challenging circumstances.

The families I worked with have remained deeply etched on my psyche all these years, although I might not have thought about them for considerable stretches of time. It feels important to have been able to share some of their stories and their poignant experiences of their illness, hospitalisation and awareness of death, especially how they impacted on their sense of self. Sebastian found a way to integrate the gift of his brother's marrow. He had to work through his fear that he might concretely merge with his brother, lose his self-other differentiation and assimilate his brother's attributes by having his bone marrow inserted and added into him. I believe his transplant was successful. He bravely fought to carry on living as full a life as possible. Akin's gift to me of the board game has needed to be described and written about, perhaps to help others learn from his experience and ways of trying to master the so-called game he had to play in his life. He knew that I understood much of what he was going through. At a moment of saying goodbye, Akin made sure that I would remember him and keep him in mind. His legacy may also be understood as a narcissistic wish to leave something of himself behind, to have made his mark. I hope that I have honoured what he bequeathed me. I learnt a great deal from my work on the ward. These two courageous young boys and their families taught me so much and helped me to face some of my own fears of death and finitude, as well as to treasure my opportunities to live as full a life as possible.

Acknowledgments

Many thanks to Edith Hargreaves and Gilbert Kliman for encouraging me to write this chapter.

William Boyd is from *From Any Human Heart* by Copyright © William Boyd 2003, 2009, published by Penguin Books 2003, 2009. Reproduced by permission of Penguin Books Ltd.

References

Bergman, T. and Freud, A. 1965. *Children in Hospital*. New York: International Universities Press.
Bluebond-Langner, M. 1978. *The Private Worlds of Dying Children*. Princeton, NJ: Princeton University Press.
Bollas, C. 1989. *Forces of Destiny*. London: Free Association Books.
Boyd, W. 2009. *Any Human Heart*. London: Penguin.
Castelnuovo-Tedesco, P. 1973. Organ Transplant, Body Image, Psychosis. *The Psychoanalytic Quarterly*, 42: 349–363.
Cohen, M. 2003. *Sent Before My Time*. London: Karnac.
Cohen, P. 1990. Coping Processes in Well-Adjusted Chronically Ill Patients on Paediatric Ward. *Journal of Child Psychotherapy*, 16(2): 39–48.
Davids, J. 2020. Reminiscences of paediatric work. Unpublished manuscript.
Elfer, J. and Lee, A. 2009. To Make a Male: What Does it Take? *Journal of Child Psychotherapy*, 35(1): 49–61.
Emmanuel, R., Colloms, A., Mendelsohn, A., Muller, H. and Testa, R. 1990. Psychotherapy with Hospitalised Children with Leukaemia: Is it Possible? *Journal of Child Psychotherapy.*, 16 (2): 21–37.

Fraiberg, S. 1982. Pathological Defences in Infancy, *Psychoanalytic Quarterly*, 51: 612–635.

Frenkel, L. 2004. "I Smile at Her and She Smiles Back at Me": Between Repair and Re-enactment: The Relationship between Nurses and Child Patients in a South African Paediatrics Burns Unit. In S. Levy and A. Lemma (Eds), *The Perversion of Loss Psychoanalytic Perspectives on Trauma*. London: Whurr.

Furman, E. 1984. Helping Children Cope with Dying. *Journal of Child Psychotherapy*, 10(2): 151–157.

Goldie, L. and Desmarais, J. 2005. *Psychotherapy and the Treatment of Cancer Patients Bearing Cancer in Mind*. London: Routledge.

Hinton, P. E. 1980. How a Ten Year Old Girl Faced Her Death. *Journal of Child Psychotherapy*, 6: 107–116.

Judd, D. 1989. *Give Sorrow Words: Working with a Dying Child*. London: Free Association Books.

Houlding, S. 2018. When a Patient Dies: Reflections on the Death of Three Patients. In C. Masur (Ed.), *Flirting with Death*. Abingdon: Routledge.

Menzies Lyth, I. 1970. The Functioning of Social Systems as a Defence against Anxiety. In I. Menzies Lyth, *Containing Anxiety in Institutions Selected Essays* (pp. 43–98). London: Free Association Books.

Moran, G. S. 1984. Psychoanalytic Treatment of Diabetic Children. *Psychoanalytic Study of the Child*, 39: 407–447.

Norton, J. 1963. The Treatment of a Dying Patient. *Psychoanalytic Study of the Child*, 18: 541–560.

Kliman, G. 1968. *Psychological Emergencies of Childhood*. New York: Grune and Stratton.

Katz, D. A. 2020. Treatment of a Dying Child. *Psychoanalytic Study of the Child*, 73 (1): 158–171.

Stern, D. N. 2004. *The Present Moment in Psychotherapy and Everyday Life*. New York: Norton.

Straker, N. (Ed.) 2013. *Facing Cancer and the Fear of Death. A Psychoanalytic Perspective on Treatment*. New York: Rowman and Littlefield.

Winnicott, D. W. 1948. Paediatrics and Psychiatry. In D. W. Winnicott, *Through Paediatrics to Psychoanalysis*. London: Hogarth.

Chapter 5

Day Hospital Intensive Care for Patients with Eating Disorders

Humberto Lorenzo Persano

Introduction

Eating disorders (ED) are a common condition today and require various and diverse interdisciplinary treatments that usually include day hospital (DH) usages. Although DH treatments are widespread, their description in the literature is limited, except for the pioneering descriptions of the Toronto (Piran et al. 1989), Munich (Gerlinghoff et al. 1998) and Turin programs (Abbate-Daga et al. 2009). There are coincidences in some aspects of them including the use of a multidisciplinary staff and support on group treatment as the primary goals of therapy. Eating DH programs also function as a transition from inpatient care to full-time life in the community and they are advantageous because partial hospitalization allows patients to maintain social and vocational roles, thus encouraging more independence (Zipfel et al. 2002).

DH for eating disorders can be divided into two types. One type is based on short-term therapeutic objectives focused on the relief of symptoms including weight recovery or ending of purgative behaviors using cognitive-behavioral frameworks. The second type of DH uses lasting therapeutic programs and focus their goals on individual functioning as well as the recovery of their abilities. These kinds of approaches are centered on the psychodynamic understanding of their symptoms as well as recovering their global functioning. They also include gradual changes in weight or behavior (Abbate-Daga et al. 2009). These DH programs are less extended than those which focus on short-term programs. Some of them use mixed programs, both psychodynamic and cognitive (Abbate-Daga et al. 2012).

Studies on the impact of DH on eating disorders are still scarce. Most of them focus on weight recovery or purging behavior changes. There is also a lack of information about psychological changes. Our experience in this field has led us to consider that we must be humble when developing theories from a single disciplinary field and this is a problem to evaluate psychological changes or treatment improvements from psychoanalytical perspectives. To this end, it is necessary to evaluate changes through psychoanalytical and extra-psychoanalytical research strategies.

DOI: 10.4324/9781003167679-6

Eating disorders and especially those considered persistent enduring eating disorders (EED), require a therapeutic approach across multiple disciplines, because each discipline by itself does not solve them, and therefore, must be carried out with an interdisciplinary and integrative approach. Dialogue among different professionals from diverse disciplines is imperative for building an integrative approach. These conditions impact not only on the real body but also on mind configuration, interpersonal relationships and personal achievements. Eating disorder patients need different perspectives from many disciplines to reach an effective treatment and a sustained outcome. We have found, through working with them and training competences and developing skills in professional teams that the psychoanalytic theoretical framework has an important place for the understanding and treatment of these clinical phenomena. The essence is not only the practice, but also deals in depth with research on the dynamics of mental functioning, self's constitution, interpersonal relationships, affect regulation, symbolization and mentalizing process (Persano 2014) as well as for developing a psychoanalytic mind (Busch 2013).

Day Hospital Intensive Care

The Day Hospital for Eating Disorders Unit at a psychiatric public hospital in Buenos Aires City is conceptually inspired by ideas developed after World War II, which emerged as a necessity to face a community mental health plan in the United Kingdom (Jones 1953). These social techniques in mental health were called the therapeutic community. The main point of this conceptual framework is to determine if the environment produce psychopathology due to disturbances among distorted human relationships. A new healthy environment could provide a new framework for psychological change and for developing healthy subjects. The environmental framework could function as an approach in therapy and has been developed as a comprehensive method for mental health treatment denominated *milieu therapie* (Ammon 1995). Our programs are designed by a two-year intensive care approach combining group and individual therapies including medical clinical control, nutritional treatment, psychoeducational food management, psychopharmacological and psychodynamic psychotherapeutic treatment. And our psychoanalytical inspired day hospital program for EED includes the environment, professional team, technical approaches, food, and commensality as well as peer's relationships in a new healthy common milieu atmosphere. These environmental factors allow new internalized object relationships, new identifications processes and would be useful for improving affect regulation.

It is important that therapeutic teams have a place during grand round sessions for discussing clinical cases, overall clinical management, group interactions and performances during the treatment process. Also, it is important supervising the clinical outcome and the psychotherapeutic process through single case supervisions. These activities are crucial for avoiding acting-out behaviors, impulsivity, and emotional arousal among patients. Transference and counter transference comprehension are also important during treatment management and psychotherapeutic process.

Psychoanalytical Contract Framework

After careful diagnostic evaluation including clinical, nutritional, psychological, psychiatric, global functioning and nursing evaluation, an inform consent and a statement based-contract are signed between the patient and the institution with the commitment to attend and fulfil rules of participation. If the patient is under 18 years old the contract is also signed by his/her parents,

From a psychoanalytical point of view, Otto Kernberg and Frank Yeomans have written about the importance of the contract-based approach for treating borderline patients (Kernberg et al. 2008; Yeomans et al. 1992). We have taken these concepts to explain the based-contract with eating disorders patients before the starting of the treatment because it functions as a frame for the therapeutical process like in classical psychoanalytic treatments and it is a supporting frame for the commitment to the treatment goals, as well as for avoiding acting-out behaviors.

Eating disorder patients have in common with personality disorder patients' similarities and most of them, mainly bulimic patients, share borderline personality organizations (BPO). We have found from statistical research identical correlations in reality testing, identity diffusion and primitive defense mechanism dimensions using The Inventory for Personality Organization (IPO) research tool (Lenzenweger 2001), and very similar in aggression and moral values dimensions both in ED samples and in BPO samples (Persano et al. 2016). These findings allow us to support the based-contract frame for day hospital program treatment. According to Frank Yeomans, and from our clinical experience, the psychodynamic day hospital approaches require the early establishment of a frame that can contain the patient's affective storms during the treatment process and also for avoiding early drop-out of it (Yeomans et al. 1994).

Specific Themes during Treatment

Main problems in patients suffering from eating disorders are conflicts between ideal and real body image. These conditions merit a prominent approach through tactics that prioritize group techniques, such as group psychotherapies and also through group thematic workshops aimed at discussing the ideals themselves in relation to those of other subjects who suffer similar conditions in a psychoanalytic theoretical framework. According to

Philippe Jeammet, anorexic patients have difficulties in the symbolization process. He metaphorically named its condition as "*anorexie mentale.*" They have a lack of representations in mind and difficulties in the appetence for the object (Jeammet 1985).

Therefore, group approaches allow them to accept from other persons listening to new words and experiences that improve the mentalizing process as well as the acceptance of new object representations in their mind. Mentalizing-based treatment is unique in focusing on enhancing the patient's capacity to think about and to regulate mental states (Fonagy & Bateman 2007).

These patients have tyrannical ideals and fanatic ideas about beauty, body shapes, body weight and appearance. We have defined the tyranny of ideals to those conflicts related between ego ideal and the ego. Patients are trapped in their own present suffering lives, and they have difficulties in talking about other themes or thinking in future projects. They suffer loneliness and in a secret way (Persano 2005). Sometimes this way of living is like living in a jail, so called by some authors as the golden cage (Bruch 2001).

The first steps of treatment focus on helping the patients release themselves from this conflict, which is associated to painful experiences and tendency to isolation and lack of interest in vital goals. Mentalizing process start from the beginning at the day hospital intensive care program through talking and listening to different experiences, interact with different personalities styles, as well as other perspectives. These tasks have a psychoanalytical conceptual framework sustained in mentalizing progressive process because it improves the symbolization process, emotional regulation, and introspection as a new way of thinking.

Although most studies focus on food or eating and body image distortion, eating disorder patients are prone to suffer from infantile traumatic experiences, distorted family functioning and sexual abuse. Frequently EED patients attempt to deal with these conflicts through compensatory behaviors to control body weight, emotional arousal or feeling of emptiness as an attempt to use these mechanisms as an omnipotent control for their frustrating or painful feelings. In addition to impulsivity and self-harming, primitive acting-out mechanisms are commonly used by the patient to deal with their unstable emotional regulation. They also are prone to depression or suicide attempts due to chronic psychic pain and mental suffering. Binge drinking, drug abuse and dysphoric affects during weekends are other common ways of functioning due to abandonment anxieties they feel when the DH is closed, and they go back to their home environment. Mondays are special days for treating these issues in group sessions. Abandonment anxieties both real and in phantasies are also commonly related to personality disorders, we have observed these manifestations mainly in bulimic patients, sometimes during weekends these patients also present some antisocial behaviors, like kleptomaniac episodes (Schwartz 1992). We have found this kind of behavior in social environment as well at the DH unit.

Although some ED patients need psychopharmacological treatment, for treating depressive symptoms, impulsivity, or symptoms of psychoticism, they also need group and individual psychotherapy, to stop acting-out behaviors and to introduce them in developing the capacity to feel their own feelings. The task is not simple since both the space and the therapeutic work time are limited and patients return to their own social and family environments as soon as they leave the therapeutic DH unit. However, our goal focuses on seeking progressive and sustained achievements within the global therapeutic atmosphere and these changes can be internalized into the mind and reinforced every week.

Thematic workshops in our program are focused on behaviors related to food and sharing lunch as well as to family conflicts and to the relationship with their sexuality and gender identity for dealing with these difficulties and conflicts. These patients have in common experiences of eating alone or within a violent family atmosphere. We have also found history of dysfunctional family patterns in these patients, like those founded in borderline family environment (Links 1990). Then family therapy and family group therapy are another aspect to approach EED patients, mainly with adolescents.

In day hospital treatments and especially in the model we are considering inspired by the psychoanalytic therapeutic unit, it is possible that individuals with severe characterological disorders can express their symptomatic constellations during their stay in the program. Affective turmoil, interpersonal conflicts, splitting images about themselves into the professional team are activations of primitive defense mechanisms and primitive internalized object relationships. Both transference and countertransference issues must be understood and must be interpreted during the therapeutic process.

The countertransference is an important diagnostic tool and allows monitoring the outcome of the psychotherapeutic process. Therefore, these affective manifestations will appear in the psychotherapeutic process during intermediate phases. As a phenomenon of intersubjective interaction, it not only occurs in dyadic situations of the analytic frame itself, but also unfolds in much more extensive situations such as those that involve the spheres of intersubjective interactions that they develop in group situations and especially in the social complexity of the day intensive care program with a therapeutic community modality. Many times, these patients arouse feelings of hatred that merit to be understood and explained during supervisions, they can lead to counteractions into the own professional team relationships (Persano 2006a). Supervisions have an important role for understanding these phenomena and for working among group and interactions with professional teams.

Intense countertransference impacts are not only due to their behaviors but also to the speech style used by these patients. In anorexic patients a monotone speech that implies a representational deficit is quite common. It is due to the difficulty to incorporate, not only food, but also preconscious mental representations. It is produced by a progressive anorexia process of mind's endowments that are translated into anorexic behavior (Jeammet 1994).

Bulimic patients, usually through affective turmoil and acting-out behaviors generate intense countertransference feelings. Their affective regulation is unstable, and they are prone to develop depressive symptoms. This difficulty can be understood as the inability to achieve certain mental states (Fonagy & Target 1996). These representational deficiencies also reach the representations of feelings, which rise the alexithymia phenomenon and implies a severe inability to express and feel feelings. I think that this inability is not only to express emotional states but also to be able to represent them, that is, to link emotions to cognitive representations, this phenomenon is observed in analytical sessions as a severe inability to express tonalities and different affective nuances. When these mental states reach consciousness, they can be expressed as their own feelings. Then they could be contained into their own mind as mental states. Many times, they appear first in the therapist as counter-transferential perceptions, and they are the pre-announcement of a psychic change (Persano 2006a).

To achieve this objective, the environment must enable the patient's capacity for introspection. This environment should allow the subject to abandon, step by step, their ties to mental suffering through progressive psychic changes and attitudes towards food, their own body images, self-esteem regulation, changes through interpersonal relationships, the way of planning their lives and how they could be included socially in a new way. It is particularly important that during the supervision processes these changes can be detected and expressed to the therapeutic team, through clinical grand rounds, clinical case presentations and psychotherapeutic evaluation process, because sometimes the own team are so involved in treating patient's symptoms and they cannot perceive these subtle changes.

Theoretical Psychoanalytical Concepts Applied to Therapeutic Process

Body image construction is a complex matter that includes no also psychological aspects but also social constructions. In the middle of the 20th century, psychoanalysis have been enriched by Paul Schilder's concepts on human body image. He postulated that the human body image is under construction during the whole life. From a dynamic point of view, the body image could be both modified by environmental and psychic factors. For this author, the body image construction is determined by the interchange of mental and social influences (Schilder 1950).

The body image and the self's constitution have close relationships with each other. Although the sense of ourselves is stable but dynamically changing through our life, some authors postulate from a neuroscientific perspective that the sense of body ownership is a fragile outcome of integrating multiple sensory signals (Tsakiris 2010, 2017).

According to Peter Fonagy, the mentalizing process is carried out during early stages of self-development and the attachment theory explains how mothers' and babies' relationships influence the mentalizing process in their babies (Fonagy 2001). On the other hand, Marianne Leuzinger-Bohleber explains how the body is influenced by the environment and how it modifies the intimate body. She also explains how the relations to the external world can develop and change embodied representations of the self itself (Leuzinger-Bohleber 2018). Therefore, the construction of the "self" and body images depends on early interactions among parental figures and the infant. Later social interactions are also significant in their construction, deconstruction and reconfiguration. These conceptualizations are crucial to understand the importance of peer groups interactions within the community DH programs.

Other aspect to understand psychodynamics of eating disorders are related to conflict theory and defense mechanism theory. There are different conflict levels and defense mechanism levels in eating disorder patients. There are patients who evidence discomfort with their body images and high ideal expectations about their bodies. These patients are more related to narcissistic personality disorders. These patients require a brief period in day intensive care programs and are capable for outpatient's unit treatment. But others who have shown distortions of their body's images, primitive defenses, and identity diffusion, as well as severe difficulties in affect regulation and impulsive behavior are related to borderline personality organizations. These patients require DH intensive care. There are others who have shown severe distorted body images, frankly psychotic like thoughts and withdrawal from reality are related to psychotic functioning. These patients require specific approaches at the day hospital intensive care. The major distortion of body's images and object's representation requires most specific treatments for recovering the ownership of their "self."

These observations from clinical practice state that eating disorders could be related to different psychopathological dimensions and personality organizations and they need specific approaches although they could be treated at the same DH unit program.

Therefore, through clinical observations in our daily task we can make some psychoanalytical theoretical understanding and allow us to understand unconscious mind configurations and mental psychodynamics functioning.

Through these observations we have found different types of problems in eating disorders patients. One of them is related to early parent–infant failed meetings (mismatches). Parents have committed neglect with their children for different reasons, but their children have the same problem with mirroring functioning, and consequently their children are not enough cathected by erotic or love narcissistic libido. These kind of mismatches among parents, mostly observed in mothers and babies, creates a failed mirroring encounter.

I have described that this phenomenon of mothers creating a failed mirroring as a "*Snow White syndrome*," where girls look at the mirror seeking for an acceptance and good feedback response, but they have found a bad image reflecting an ugly image of themselves, like a witch (Persano 2005). Then they identify with this ugly image of themselves and they think that beauty is in other girls but not in themselves. This conflict persists in any kind of relationship and in any kind of mirror images from the external world provided by culture. The mirror introduces us to the so-called clinic of the gaze.

For Paulina Kernberg, the mirror represents the image of the mother and the infant relates to it. The infant relates to mirror as her/his own mother, the mirror is an equivalent of her (Kernberg 1984, 1987). The recognition of the infant in the mirror awakens an emotion of joy at her/his discovery as an integrated human being. The role of mirrors is to convey projectively children's relationships with their mothers as well as their own sense of self (Kernberg et al. 2007). The mirror at present is represented through the multiplicity of maddening images that are provided by the great diffusion that our culture makes possible and repeats, over and over again, that beauty is in another place less in ourselves. By its virtual features, this reality is elusive. This identification with cruelty is responsible for the mistreatment of the real body, in many patients as if they were someone else's, and therefore, they never find peace and approval.

The desired and idealized body image is always too far from the representation of their own real body and they fail in transforming body's sensations into pleasant experiences, because these are unknown to them. The tyranny of aesthetic ideals prevails over bodily sensations and erotic gratification.

The mirror represents, then, a lackluster image of the person, despite belonging to the so-called narcissistic pathologies, they differ significantly from the myth of Narcissus, since girls do not fall in love with their own image but feel a deep contempt for it. Eating disorder patients live totally dependent on the mirror, they unsuccessfully seek the approval of the mirror, but paradoxically it gives them back an unpleasant look at themselves, which is due to deep primitive projections of denigrated aspects of the self (Persano 2005).

These young women are extremely demanding and extremely dependent on projected images by the prevailing models in our culture. They run after those alien images. The mirror returns a distorted message that seems to announce that they will never reflect a beautiful image of themselves. In trying to achieve this, they alienate themselves and ignore their own body, they treat it as if it is not real, as if it is a simple image. Revenge now turns against the subject himself, in a feeling of infinite hatred. The idealized image is so distorted that it is now transformed into a frantic and real search for themselves; unknowing their own real body, they almost acquire an eidetic essence of the "self." The image with which they have primarily identified becomes an early constitution of the primitive ego ideal, and it is more invested by aggression than by libido (Persano 2005).

Although the sense of ourselves is a fragile outcome of integrating multiple sensory signals, in both, the brain in the neurosciences and the mind in psychoanalytic mind's theory, our inner world has a relative stable representation. But in ED patients, the conflict between body's images and the "self" construction is very primitive, and it occurs while body's representation is under construction. Without any kind of therapeutic intervention, this conflict will last for long periods of time. Therefore, ED patients need a stable therapeutic frame during long periods at the DH intensive care program for unfolding the conflict.

Other kind of problems that we frequently observe is when these girls have suffered from physical and sexual abuse. These girls have severe difficulties in integrating their body images with loving narcissistic libido as well as severe difficulties to integrate loving or positive affects with their object relationships. In these cases, the self is embodied with aggression from the early stages of life. They feel empty and depressed, and they cannot integrate their own body images in a positive way. For Andre Green (1980), the mental emptiness clinic is determined by defensive mechanisms that are organized around withdrawal, both from the representational world and the affects' world.

Patients are trapped in this type of archaic mental functioning and they repeat in the transference the feelings of emptiness and deep loneliness, as well as depressive characterological symptoms. These types of depressive symptoms are very common to observe in patients with eating disorders, they are part of the characterological depressions, which in general do not respond adequately to pharmacological treatment with antidepressant because the symptoms are deeply immersed into their personality structure.

Sydney Blatt mentions that in anaclitic depression the mental representation of the object is altered due to an emotional withdrawal reaction. Children being alone or confronted with a stranger present muscular inactivity, hypotonia, sad facial expression, decreased gastric secretion and eventually sleep states (Blatt 1974, 2004). These characteristics are frequently observed in EED patients, which reinforce the hypothesis of defensive withdrawal and severe disturbances in the symbolization processes that give rise to the establishment of an essential depression and manifested clinically as feelings of emptiness, boredom accompanied by lethargy and alexithymia (Persano 2005).

Some authors have recently described a strong relationship between insecure anxious attachment patterns and lower self-esteem, suggesting that concerns about body image are related to insecure attachment patterns, disturbed affective regulation and alexithymia (Keating et al. 2013). Some authors have founded that high attachment anxieties predict poor outcome from cognitive-behavioral therapies (CBT) but good outcomes for psychodynamic psychotherapies. An avoidant attachment predicts less early engagement in treatment and then poor outcomes (Thompson-Brenner & Richards 2017). All these issues are expressed in everyday life at the DH intensive care.

During regressive conditions, these patients like to refuge in autistic phantasies to disappear from the real world. The embodied self with aggression is prone to commit suicide or address aggression against the own self. Multi-impulsive behaviors, and alcohol and substance abuse are attempts to avoid painful feelings; these girls are at extreme risk. They have embodiment of traumatic events, then the body becomes as an external object which could be destroyed. Specific frameworks for containing these painful emotions are a challenge in our program.

Intensive care DH is also crucial for approaching these kinds of problems due to the complexity of these conditions and the imperative need for an interdisciplinary approach from different therapeutic perspectives. Usually primitive mind functioning, acting-out behaviors, splitting defense mechanism phenomena are expressed through enactment behaviors and through the transference phenomenon into the professional team. During the psychotherapeutic process integration of different self-representations and object representations occur into the setting of the DH program. Then patients are capable to accept and integrate progressively these representations into their minds. It is a not an easy process and time and expertise are needed to conduct this kind of treatments.

The Feminine

Eating disorders are dominant in women, 90% of those affected being female, and only 10% male, mainly in adolescents. Adolescence is a challenging time for body image configuration because dramatic events happen, both in the real body as well as in the imaginary, symbolic and erotic body dimensions. Females' adolescence is more challenging than men's adolescence because they move faster from girls to women than boys do to men (Persano 2018). Their bodies are being transformed and metamorphosed by powerful inner drives in addition of interacting with a changing real external world. Most theories emphasize the cultural aspects of fashion and their relationship with eating disorders. However, in our experience with EED, we found severe mismatches at an early stage of body image construction that damages the female's body representation. By the reconstruction through psychodynamic therapy, we have also found severe aggressive attacks from mothers and fathers against the incipient female body image construction in girls. The body image construction is also damaged by sexual abuse both in girls and little boys. These aggressive attacks to the incipient self and body images construction are linked to self-harming behaviors and suicidal attempts later during adolescence or youthhood. The more severe the early traumatic experiences occur, the more severe are the eating disorders conditions observed later in life.

These severe conditions that occur in EED patients are linked to severe personality disorders, depressive symptoms and substance abuse behaviors. In clinical settings, we have found that they have difficulties in keeping a positive body image of themselves and they commonly suffer from dysregulation of affects and disturbing behaviors. Consequently, their self-esteem is very damaged, which is linked also to suicidal attempts or self-harming behaviors. Also, when an impulsive behavior is a dominant affective state, aggression also turns against themselves and behaviors like self-harming or suicides attempts are frequently exhibited. These girls have problems in thinking and feeling. The representational world is also damaged and mentalizing process fails. Acting-out and major distorting defense mechanisms are frequently observed in their speech and their behavior.

During the adolescent process, these kinds of painful experiences become more vivid as these girls have difficulties in symbolization and mentalizing processes and they feel pain on their bodies, but they cannot feel painful experiences in their minds. They have hatred object relationships internalized, and thereafter, their own condition become worsts. They externalize this inner world into the external relationship world. Failure in mirroring process also affect self-esteem and affect's the regulation as well as the identity constitution process. The construction of the feminine identity is also damaged or disturbed. New interactions and new interpersonal relationships at the DH environment help them to deconstruct these damages into the feminine and to rebuild new inner world configurations.

Mentalizing and Embodiment Experiences at Day Hospital Intensive Care

From this perspective, we can observe the intrinsic relationship between mentalizing process and the embodiment experiences interacting with each other. However, embodiment experiences cannot be changed by the representational world changing process, as is the case in psychoanalysis "on the couch" works. These embodied memories need new embodiment experiences to be integrated and rebuilt. Consequently, new experiences through new healthy interpersonal relationships, as well as healthy new environmental experiences that occur during psychoanalytic "out of the couch" day hospital treatment programs are important for the therapeutic process.

The understanding of mentalizing process theory allows us to comprehend some intrinsic circumstances of eating disorder patients. For Peter Fonagy, eating disorder patients have severe difficulties in the mentalizing process.

This is particularly important in anorexic patients. These patients are prone to feel sensations in their real bodies rather than feelings on their minding bodies about themselves. Fonagy agrees that ED patients have in common severe difficulties in expressing themselves in terms of thinking, feeling, or perceiving their own mental states.

This lack of mentalization that has been originated at an early stage of life is related to difficulties in the attachment process, and therefore, in the symbolization process and in the representations of themselves configuration. They experience bodily sensations more than mental states. Patients can state that the distortion of their body image is a strong sensation related to negative affects like fear, anger or sadness, but these feelings are felt in their own body rather than in mental states (Skårderud & Fonagy 2012).

The body takes and excessive central role in the continuity of the sense of self. Or we can observe this lacking mentalizing process when they do not have a clear sense of themselves and need a sense of themselves according to how other people react to them. Usually, they use to treat themselves as objects, but not metaphorically because the self is experienced as a physical object without a clear psychological meaning (Fonagy et al. 2002).

I think this point of view is shared with Philippe Jeammet, but for him this process is not a deterioration of the symbolization process, but rather an active way of withdrawal from reality as a defensive mechanism. These patients have a primitive reaction to defend themself against their own body image perception that includes withdrawing affect from representations, and therefore, the symbolization process is deteriorated (Jeammet 1985). Jeammet stablished that these types of disorders belong to psychosomatic pathology, that is, early failures in the structuring of the self (*Moi*) that disturb personality structure development (ibid.).

Because this occurs at an early stage of the child's development, the attachment pattern and the feeding process are compromised. This occurs because the latter is established by a bonding modality, and because of the early mismatches, the attachment patterns are altered as well as the emotional regulatory system and the feeding process (Persano 2006b).

We have found that distortions in body image is a constant not only in anorexic patients but also in bulimic patients (Persano et al. 2019). In a recent pilot study, we have found that distortion in object perception is also observed more frequently than the distortion in the body image and self-representation (Gutnisky et al. 2019). These findings allow us to hypothesize that distortions of both object's representation into the inner world as self-representations are constant in these patients. Therefore, they show persistent difficulties in how they perceive themselves and other people. And probably these misperceptions are related to very distorted primitive object relationships internalized during early infancy. This is important for the psychotherapeutic process because we need to be remarkably close to misperceptions of our intervention's during the psychotherapeutic process.

These misperceptions are expressed both, during the therapeutical processes and during formation of new interpersonal relationships at the day hospital. The patients need a long period of time to internalize new perceptions of themselves, provided by the therapeutical environment of the day hospital intensive care and from the psychotherapeutic process itself. These changes occur not only into the mind of the individual but also in brain networks, and therefore, the changes also reconfigure intersubjective brain networks. For mentalization-based treatment (MBT) of eating disorder patients the main goal is not to content but "minding the minds as a competence." The concept "embodied mentalizing" implies that the body fill in the mentalizing failure, because they are hyper-embodied in sensations, but at the same time they are disembodied in mentalizing and feelings (Skårderud & Fonagy 2012).

As it occurs in transference focused psychotherapy (TFP) (Kernberg et al. 2008) it is important that their failure in the mentalization process could be interpreted here and now during the therapeutic encounters. Then transference is a significative concept to consider in these therapeutic processes during psychoanalysis out of couch approach.

In our eating disorders intensive care day hospital program, patients can make an embodiment of positive affect experiences that allows the mentalizing process to arise. Mentalizing and embodiment process interact in a positive way and allow enduring psychic changes.

Why Day Hospital Intensive Care with a Psychoanalytic Framework?

Out of the couch psychoanalysis can be carried out in mental health units for people who suffer from severe traumatized experiences that occur in their early infancy and that are manifested later in life as psychopathological conditions. We need to conceptualize a clear framework for applying psychoanalytic approaches in a public hospital day intensive care for eating disorders.

Psychoanalysis is a discipline that encourages patients to be committed to a deep knowledge of the genesis of their own suffering, and at the same time, it requires that the patients also are an active and responsible participant in the healing process. Any attempt that keeps patients alienated from the reason for their own suffering and that tries to demonstrate an image of absolute efficacy, outside of patients themselves, is highly likely to fail. For this same reason, treating EED patients by unique individual psychotherapy approach could also fail when the causes are extraordinarily complex. Therefore, an interdisciplinary approach is extremely important for treating EED patients.

These failures are due to the very characteristics of the hypermodern individual, following the ideas of Marcel Gauchet who calls this phenomenon as "excessive individualism." He writes as antithesis way the structuring of a "collective reality" or of a "social space," called the "collective operation" (*le fonctionnement collectif*; Rothnie 1994). But in our society one individual could have the exclusivity of being the first individual to live ignoring that he/she lives in a society. It could also be the first individual who can allow him/herself to ignore that they live in society due to the very evolution of society itself (Castel 2009). To be able to work in a therapeutic community program, one must allow oneself to discard individualistic ties to one's own discipline, which are inevitable and are promoted by the type of academic training that each health professional receives, to co-think and cooperate through interdisciplinary and complementary approaches.

A risk of individual-focused treatments is that these approaches comply with manifestations of postmodernity societies, in which individualism prevails (Lipovetsky 1983). Individual treatments are transformed into spaces that can repeat the tension between two perspectives. One of them, is that patients suffer in their own isolation as a consequence of their own fanatic idealized values, and the other, is the subject in the role of a health professional who tries to solve the condition with his/her own therapeutic resources learned in the individualistic scenario of each discipline. To approach these problems exclusively in the individual field of psychotherapy or the nutritional therapy, or the psychopharmacological approach is exceedingly difficult due to reductionism and limits of each discipline.

These disorders become intrinsic characterological features of an ego-syntonic nature and they are not perceived as a disease by those who suffer from them, sometimes they believe that is a way of living. Both, patient's isolation and therapeutic individualism, are serious challenge for treating ED patients. We are working at the frontiers of each discipline and it is mandatory to work in an interdisciplinary environment to put in practice these different perspectives.

We agree to what Racamier calls the work of the psychoanalyst without a couch, to explain his work in the field of healthcare institutions (Racamier 1970). This concept is extremely useful in our daily practice from which many people benefit, not only patients but also professionals in the health field who enjoy and learn from shared teamwork. Those who are in the formative stage since the beginning they apprehend the co-thinking experience in a collective program from an interdisciplinary viewpoint and prone to dialogue among different colleagues with diverse knowledge but working together with same goal. This viewpoint is intrinsically psychoanalytic because listening to others is the main goal, although we are not working through an individual psychotherapy approach. Understanding different points of view and other perspectives is also related to create a psychoanalytic mind, but a collective one. Patients improve also from sharing different perspectives and interventions about their own suffering.

Another last issue, but not less important in promoting public policy in health, is to develop models inspired by the psychodynamic therapeutic community, because they are particularly useful when applied in the public sphere, since they allow reaching a larger number of patients and promote free and equal access to the right to mental health. It is a great contribution of psychoanalysis to the community.

In day hospital treatments, and especially in the therapeutic community model that we are proposing, patients with severe characterological disorders express their symptomatic constellations and they are contained in the frame of these psychodynamic approaches. Due to the transference phenomenon, they not only activate their primitive object relations at the intrapsychic level, but also at the interpersonal level in everyday treatment programs. The neutrality of the team is essential to be able to understand the psychodynamics of the process. In addition, especially useful the use of the transference phenomenon to understand and interpret their symptoms and behaviors (Kernberg 1977).

A central aspect of any day hospital intensive care program unit is constituted by the day living workshops where a dialogue is made about the difficulties of the group, in the daily living together in the day hospital, with the purpose of moving from the intolerance of other ideas or other perspectives towards the acceptance of intersubjective differences. Therapeutic groups try to transform patient's isolation condition into bonding experience as well solidarity towards the other participants and thus build the notion of groupness. Through weekly sessions carried out in small groups, patients can display their sufferings in a more private environment and therapists can use more interpretive interventions than in workshops. Thematic workshops aim to reconsider values and ideals in order to abandon the tyranny of them, within the framework of a group with therapeutic objectives and with the possibility that each group's member can be mirrored in another peer to internalize new representations into the inner world.

It is important to highlight than during lunch both professional staff members and patients should eat together. The sharing of this space improves commensality, food habits and it is also humanizing. Therefore, the dining room plays an important role as a milieu with a therapeutic atmosphere. The main goal is that patients stop eating in secret and experience sharing a lunch. These patients use to eat alone, in secret or in family hostile environments and they have lost the notion of what commensality means. This therapeutic environment helps to monitor the eating plan and to modify food habits, while simultaneously enabling human interactions and rescuing the role of commensality in human beings, which is commonly forgotten in our society but is now rescued in the psychodynamic therapeutic community day hospital unit program.

The main goal of all these therapeutic approaches is improving patient's functioning into a global treatment strategy. Psychic change can be summarized as the passage from suffering to enjoy living, and this is a deep transformation of their own's lives.

When Introduce Individual Psychodynamic Psychotherapy?

Partial hospitalization units with psychodynamic therapeutic model allow patients to begin to construct their own narratives through different group interventions that increase the capacity for representability and symbolization as well as for the historization process. At more advanced steps, day hospital intensive care treatment patients usually ask for individual psychotherapy treatment. This demand is important by itself because patients move from ego syntonic symptoms to feel anguish and wishes of being helped. These feelings announce psychic changes. Because they move from primitive defensive functioning as acting out, splitting, withdrawal from reality, idealization or devaluation and omnipotence, to show ways of the emergence of higher-level defensive mechanisms including affiliation, which is manifested through asking for help. Seeking for help implies the abandon of the omnipotent control and the abandon of a protective shell in suffering in isolation. These patients are asking for more privately psychotherapeutic encounters, which represents a positive change. They are looking forward to a change in their way of living.

When patients reach this point of the treatment, a progressive process of transition from the day hospital intensive care to a less frequency modality. They move from five to three days a week and they can return to partial school or social activities. If the outcomes are functioning well, then they are discharged from the day hospital and admitted introduced into an outpatient's program at the same unit. In our approach, this a special moment to introduce patients to individual psychotherapy.

The psychotherapeutic process is a hard work. During this process, archaic psychic functioning remains active, which is also linked to the presence of primitive mental contents. This phenomenon not only obeys a regressive and defensive dynamic but also shows the type of archaic mental structure. Individual psychodynamic psychotherapy is like an open door, a challenge for change but it is also an opportunity for making enduring psychic changes.

In this sense, the first phases of psychotherapeutic treatment, with this type of patient, implies that the therapist can tolerate these primitive transference manifestations and expose them to the patient, since patients lack the reflective capacity about their own archaic mental functioning. Psychoanalytic psychotherapy is a specific indication for this type of disturbance and requires an active role on the part of the therapist, since the technique of conventional psychoanalysis is useful for approaching neuroses, but is not well tolerated by patients with archaic mental functioning. Especially, they do not tolerate prolonged silences because they awaken intense feelings of loneliness and abandonment. They activate the most primitive defensive responses that tend to perpetuate the psychopathological circle. But psychotherapeutic process shows progress, and then subtle intrapsychic transformations and psychic change are possible. Especially, they show changes in nuances of humor, defensive style functioning, interpersonal relationships, and it is related to changes not only in the inner world but also in the outer world, because manifestations in vocational attitudes, desires, projects and love relationships emerge.

We consider that to carry out individual psychotherapy in hospital environments it is appropriate to use manualized psychoanalytic psychotherapies like transference focus psychotherapy (TFP; Kernberg et al. 2008) or mentalization based treatment (MBT; Allen & Fonagy 2006). We use both MBT at early stages of treatments during day hospital treatment as well as during early stages at ambulatory treatments and TFP when patients are capable for understanding clarifications, confrontations, or interpretations during the psychotherapeutic process. According to our clinical observations, MBT is useful in anorexic patients while TFP functions better in bulimic patients with borderline personality organizations. But we need more empirical studies to affirm our clinical observations.

Manualized psychoanalytic psychotherapies are also useful for training residents in the mental health field. They have clear strategies, tactics and technical approaches during different phases of the treatment. Residents in the mental health field interested in psychodynamic treatments could benefit from these approaches. Manualized psychodynamic psychotherapies have in common global treatment strategies, which imply promoting mentalizing and symbolization process by the MBT mode, and the integration of splitting self and objects representations, which rescue the subject from the fragmentation of their identity diffusion by TFP model.

By promoting psychic integration and mentalizing process, patients take over their body new embodiment experiences, and their own thoughts acquire a stabilization in their psychic organization. This phase of the treatment is intended to facilitate the processing of conflicts in the psychic sphere and allows patients, in a more advanced phase of the psychotherapeutic process, to free themselves from extreme dependence on the gaze of others and from the tyranny of their own ethical and aesthetic ideals. They can then progressively take over the sensations of their own body and recognize their complex world of emotions. Finally, they can change their way of painful living for a more pleasant life.

References

Abbate-Daga, G., Gramaglia, C., Preda, S., Comba, E., Brustolin, A. & Fassino, S. (2009). Day hospital programmes for eating disorders: a review of the similarities, differences, and goals. *Eating and Weight Disorders*, 14(2–3), e31–e41.

Abbate-Daga, G., Gramaglia, C., Panero, M., De Bacco, C., Brustolin, A., Campisi, S., Marzola, E., Quaranta, M., Buzzichelli, S., Notaro, G. & Fassino, S. (2012). Il Trattamento dei disturbi del comportamento alimentari nel day hospital psichiatrico. *Dati preliminari. Minerva Psychiat.* 53, 1–10.

Allen, J.G. & Fonagy, P. (Eds.) (2006). *The handbook of mentalization-based treatment*. Chichester: John Wiley & Sons.

Ammon, G. (1995). Theoretical aspects of milieu therapy. *Dynamische Psychiatrie, Int. Zeischrift Fûr Psychiatrie Und Psychoanalyse*, 3(6), 282–311.

Blatt, S. (1974). Levels of object representation in anaclitic and introjective depression. *Psychoanal. Stud. of Child*, 29, 107–157.

Blatt, S. (2004). *Experiences of depression: Theoretical clinical and research perspectives*. Washington, DC: American Psychological Association.

Bruch, H. (2001). *The golden cage: The enigma of anorexia nervosa*. Boston, MA: Harvard University Press.

Busch, F. (2013). *Creating a psychoanalytic mind: A psychoanalytic method and theory*. London: Routledge.

Castel, R. (2009). *El ascenso de las incertidumbres: Trabajo, protecciones, estatuto del individuo*. Buenos Aires: Ed. Fondo de Cultura Económica, Sociología.

Fonagy, P. (2001). *Attachment theory and psychoanalysis*. New York: Other Press.

Fonagy, P. & Target, M. (1996). Playing with reality: I. Theory of mind and the normal development of psychic reality. *International Journal Psychoanalysis.*, 77, 217–233.

Fonagy, P., Jurist, G. & Target, M. (2002). *Affect regulation, mentalization, and the development of the self*. New York: Other Press.

Fonagy, P. & Bateman, A.W. (2007). Mentalizing and borderline personality disorder. *Journal of Mental Health*, 16(1), 83–101.

Gerlinghoff, M., Backmund, H. & Franzen, U. (1998). Evaluation of a day treatment program for eating disorders. *Eur. Eat. Disord.*, 6, 6–106.

Green, A. (1980). *Narcisismo de vida, narcisismo de muerte*. Buenos Aires: Amorrortu Editores.

Gutnisky, D., Persano, H. & Campos, D. (2019). *Food size distortion in eating disorders: Development of a simple photographic test*. RC Psych International Congress, London, July.

Jeammet, P. (1985). L'Anorexie mentale. *Encycl. Med. Chir. Psychiatrie*, 37350, A10–A15.

Jeammet, P. (1994). El abordaje psicoanalítico de los trastornos de las conductas alimentarias. *Psicoanálisis con Niños y Adolescentes*, 6, 25–42.

Jones, M. (1953). *The therapeutic community: a new treatment method in psychiatry*. New York, Basic Books.

Keating, L., Tasca, G.A. & Hill, R. (2013). Structural relationships among attachment insecurity, alexithymia, and body esteem in women with eating disorders. *Eating Behaviors*, 14(3), 366–373.

Kernberg, O.F. (1977). Hacia una teoría integral del tratamiento hospitalario. In *La Teoría de las relaciones Objetales y el Psicoanálisis Clínico*. Buenos Aires: Ed. Paidós.

Kernberg, O.F., Yeomans, F.E., Clarkin, J.F. & Levy, K.N. (2008). Transference focused psychotherapy: Overview and update. *The International Journal of Psychoanalysis*, 89(3), 601–620.

Kernberg, P.F. (1984). Reflections in the mirror: Mother–child interactions, self-awareness, and self-recognition. In J.D. Call, E. Galenson & R.L. Tyson (Eds.), *Frontiers of infant psychiatry*, vol. 2, 101–110. New York: Basic Books.

Kernberg, P.F. (1987). Mother-child interaction and mirror behavior. *Infant Mental Health Journal* 8(4), 329–339.

Kernberg, P.F., Buhl-Nielsen, B. & Normandin, L. (2007). *Beyond the reflection: The role of the mirror paradigm in clinical practice*. New York: Other Press.

Lenzenweger, M.F., Clarkin, J. F., Kernberg, O.F. & Foelsch, P.A. (2001). The Inventory of Personality Organization: Psychometric properties, factorial composition, and criterion relations with affect, aggressive dyscontrol, psychosis proneness, and self-domains in a nonclinical sample. *Psychological Assessment*, 13(4), 577.

Leuzinger-Bohleber, M. (2018). *Finding the Body in the Mind: Embodied memories, trauma, and depression*. New York: Routledge, 2018.

Links, P.S. (Ed.). (1990). *Family environment and borderline personality disorder*. Arlington, VA: American Psychiatric Association.

Lipovetsky, G. (1983). *La Era del Vacío: Ensayos sobre el individualismo contemporáneo*. Barcelona: Ed. Anagrama, Colección Compactos.

Persano, H.L. (2005). Abordajem psicodinâmica do paciente com transtornos alimentares. In C. Eizirik, R. Aguiar & S. Schestatsky (Eds.), *Psicoterapia de Orientação Analítica*, 674–688. Porto Alegre: Artmed Editora.

Persano, H.L. (2006a): Contratransferência em pacientes com transtornos alimentares. In J. Zaslavsky & M. Pires dos Santos (Eds.), *Contratransferência: teoria e prática clínica*, 150–166. Porto Alegre: Artmed Editora.

Persano, H.L. (2006b): La importancia de la Teoría del Apego en la Nutrición Infantil. *Revista DIAETA de la Asociación Argentina de Dietistas y Nutricionistas Dietistas* 24(114), 24–34.

Persano, H. (2014). El Hospital de Día para Sujetos con Trastornos de la Conducta Alimentaria: Abordaje interdisciplinario en comunidad terapéutica con enfoque psicodinámico. *PROAPSI Programa de Actualización en Psiquiatría* 3(1), 129–168.

Persano, H. (2018). Las Transformaciones Puberales y Adolescentes. In *El mundo de la salud mental en la práctica clínica*, Capítulo 18, 221–240. Buenos Aires: Ed. Akadia.

Persano, H., Gutnisky, D. & Ventura, A. (2016). *The inventory of personality organization (IPO) in clinical (BPD-ED) and control samples*. 9th Joseph Sandler Conference, Buenos Aires, Argentina, June.

Persano, H., Ciccioli, M., Gonzalo, M., Jubany, F.A., Pugliese, C.S. & Soto S. (2019). Ansiedad y trastornos de la conducta: Estudio empírico sobre una muestra clínica y un grupo control. *Rev. Nutrición Investiga*, IV(2), 154–194.

Piran N., Kaplan A., Kerr A., Shekter-Wolfson L., Winocur J., Gold E., Garfinkel, P. E. (1989). A day hospital program for anorexia and bulimia. *International Journal of Eating Disorders*, 8, 511–521.

Racamier, P.C. (1970). *Le Psychanalyste sans divan*. Paris: Ed. Puyot.

Rothnie, S. (1994). The democratic malaise: An interview with Marcel Gauchet. *Thesis Eleven*, 38(1), 138–157.

Schilder, P. (1950). *The image and appearance of the human body: Studies in the constructive energies of the psyche*. London: Routledge, 1999.

Schwartz, H.J. (1992). Psychoanalytic psychotherapy for a woman with diagnoses of kleptomania and bulimia. *Psychiatric Services*, 43(2), 109–110.

Skårderud, F. & Fonagy, P. (2012). Eating disorders. In A.W. Bateman & P. Fonagy (Eds.), *Handbook of mentalizing in mental health practice*, 347–383. Arlington, VA: American Psychiatric Association Publishing.

Thompson-Brenner, H. & Richards, L.K. (2015). Eating disorders. In P. Luyten, L.C. Mayes, P. Fonagy, M. Target & S. Blatt (Eds.), *Handbook of psychodynamic approaches to psychopathology*, 234–258, New York: The Guilford Press.

Tsakiris, M. (2010). My body in the brain: a neurocognitive model of body-ownership. *Neuropsychologia*, 48(3), 703–712.
Tsakiris, M. (2017). The multisensory basis of the self: from body to identity to others. *The Quarterly Journal of Experimental Psychology*, 70(4), 597–609.
Yeomans, F.E., Selzer, M.A. & Clarkin, J.F. (1992). *Treating the borderline patient: A contract-based approach*. New York: Basic Books.
Yeomans, F., Gutfreund, J., Selzer, M., Clarkin, J., Hull, J. & Smith, T. (1994). Factors related to drop-outs by borderline patients: Treatment contract and therapeutic alliance. *The Journal of Psychotherapy Practice and Research*, 3(1), 16.
Zipfel, S. et al. (2002). Day hospitalization programs for eating disorders: A systematic review of the literature. *International Journal of Eating Disorders*, 31(2), 105–117.

Chapter 6

Eating Disorders in Childhood and Adolescence

An Interdisciplinary Approach

Monica Zac, Sandra Novas, Luz María Zappa, Julian Onaindia, Alejandra Ariovich and Andrea Fränkel

Introduction

In this chapter, we will try to show how psychoanalytic thought can be applied in interdisciplinary work with severe pathologies in children and adolescents. We will describe the way in which we deal with one of the frequent pathologies in children and adolescents: severe eating disorders that require hospitalization.

In this chapter, we are going to share historical facts of the Unit of Mental Health at the Children General Hospital "Ricardo Gutiérrez." Such facts are intertwined with the history of our country and, therefore, with the history of our patients and ours.

As psychoanalysts, we consider that the history and the process of historization are foundational in the constitution of the psychic apparatus.

Definitions

Anorexia nervosa is considered by the World Health Organization (WHO) as a disorder characterized by the presence of a deliberate loss of weight, induced or maintained by the patient himself. It is a mental illness derived from an intense fear of obesity, in which the person generates a series of behaviors that aim to achieve the ideal of the perfect body.

Anorexia, as a mental illness with direct somatic repercussions of a strong psychic determination, occurs today in a large number of adolescents, especially women, generally in moments close to menarche, or after it. As a symptom, anorexia is found in boys and girls from babies to puberty, with different relations physical and hormonal development. In fact, it can also be manifested in early puberty, with characteristics similar to adolescents.

This illness, which affects behavior and habit related to eating, is a testimony of the suffering and disorganization of the self and at the same time represents an attempt at rearrangement. The symptoms manifested by the patients show us are emotional problems that play a role in the psychic dynamics and in the balance of the personality.

DOI: 10.4324/9781003167679-7

It would be reductionist to understand an illness of such complexity only in relation to eating and food. According to Jeammet (1994), anorexia nervosa can be understood as a set of symptoms and signs that condense meanings that will be found throughout therapeutic work. Throughout psychoanalytic literature there have been different psychopathological understandings of anorexia.

In working with adolescents we need flexibility to establish a good link with the patient and flexibility to understand the underlying structure and make a diagnosis. We must also take into account the need adolescents have to play different roles and identifications. Therefore, it is possible that many adolescents' manifestations are not the product of a specific psychic structure.

In some patients, refusal to eat can be the result of a phobic, hysterical, depressive or psychotic symptom. Only when we can find fantasies and myths behind these behaviors, they have the status of a symptom. It is a solution that the psyche finds between what is desired and what is forbidden, it predominates in neuroses. When the intrapsychic conflict is not present, we consider them as disorders. In such cases, there is no symbolic capacity and it appears as an act that has no possibility of being controlled, with a psychic apparatus that has flaws in its constitution. Such manifestations predominate in narcissistic pathologies.

In certain cases the refusal to eat is a way of seeking active opposition to the adult. It is related to the need to confront present in any normal adolescent that seeks growth. However, the irreducible refusal to eat, putting life at risk, is a "no" that does not contribute to the construction of subjectivity. It predominates in adolescents with narcissistic disorders and / or psychosis.

According to Massimo Recalcatti (2011) the anorexia–bulimia discourse can be seen in different psychic structures. It consists of a maneuver of the subject to place a barrier with respect to the devourer Other in the case of psychosis or a provocation directed at the Other in the case of neurosis. The irreducible refusal to eat, putting life at risk, is a "no" that does not contribute to the construction of subjectivity. It predominates in adolescents with narcissistic disorders and/or psychosis.

Anorexia and Family

Many works have been written about the importance of the role of the family in the development and in the treatment of mental illness. Therefore we have to ask ourselves about the relationship between the family and a child or in this case an adolescent who is suffering from anorexia nervosa. It is important to understand if the family can help their children in the complex process of growing.

In relation to the family's profile, Kestemberg (1976) describes one of the maternal profiles of the mothers of patients with anorexia as "extremely giving, perfectionist mothers." She says that they are mothers attentive to the needs of each member of the family, and perfectionists, they show an inhibition in the expression of their own needs. The mother communicates an ideal of the feminine. However, she ALSO mentions the existence of irritability and unexpressed resentment, especially in the marital relationship.

On the other hand, Minuchin (1978) shows in his study that the family system has interactive and organizational models with dysfunctional characteristics. These characteristics are the following: (1) agglutination, (2) overprotection, (3) rigidity, (4) lack of conflict resolution, and (5) the child involved in the parental conflict.

We consider it beneficial to include and involve the whole family in the treatment of this disease, given the dysfunctional modality in the establishments of its links. The family environment, the home, is the social and physical environment where meals are made and socialized. Meals follow familiar rites, habits and norms. This is because food has an important emotional component in the family environment. Indeed, parents in general, have attributed and assumed, even before the start of their duties, their role as feeders.

Then we must, through an adequate and exhaustive diagnosis, know the dynamics and characteristics of the family's functioning. The treatment can be more effective when the family is part of it and not only addressed to the patient's conflict. In most cases, we can verify that it can also be useful for the rest of the members of the family.

It is important that we help them to solve family conflicts inherent to the origin of this condition, to the repercussions once the disease is installed or to build the necessary alliance between the treating team and the family. This work with the family as part of the psychological treatment should always include the interdisciplinary work in the treatment of the eating disorders as part of the psychological treatment.

Dynamic Psychiatry

Psychiatric assessment is a part of the multidisciplinary approach in eating disorders. It is a process that includes several interviews with the patient and his caregiver, where data on current symptoms and their antecedents are collected, as well as pregnancy and development history in order to build diagnostic hypotheses to guide our treatment.

It is important to determine if the eating problems are an eating disorder or if they are symptoms of some other psychopathology, such as depression or personality disorder. On the other hand, eating disorders frequently co-occur with other mental health problems, particularly anxiety disorders and depression. Determining this is important if we plan to include pharmacological treatment.

Another issue that we must always assess is suicide risk. Eating disorders, particularly anorexia nervosa, are associated with high suicide rates, being suicide the cause of 20–50% of death in these cases. We have seen this, especially in situations of refeeding.

Puberty and adolescence are undoubtedly the main triggers (Mitchison et al., 2014). Young people simultaneously experience the challenge of living with a changing and growing body, new hormone-driven impulses, new cultural expectations, sexual, intellectual and social demands, and the need to process all this with a brain that is anatomical and chemically in a state of rapid and constant changes.

Although the strategies to be adopted will be different according to the subtype of disorder in question, some lines of treatment may be quite similar.

Confidence in their own beliefs, in relation to their body image or weight, among patients suffering from anorexia nervosa, will make treatment difficult and tortuous. On the other hand, people with bulimia nervosa are characterized by rigid convictions about good and bad food that can be incorporated or should be expelled by vomiting. This rigidity of mind offers no less difficulties.

That is why it is essential to establish a firm therapeutic alliance where the disqualification of feelings and experiences of patients is avoided, and knowing that trying to modify eating behaviors through advice or arguments will only increase resistance to the proposed treatment.

It is necessary to show respect and concern for the condition of patients in all its aspects, even those that have brought them to the current state, without abandoning the intention of helping them to face difficulties that they cannot yet understand. However, it is common for patients to put themselves in the position of "masters of knowledge" while rejecting and fighting the comments of the therapists. Therefore, it will be necessary to persist without being discouraged by the patient's efforts to defeat any attempt to help them.

We consider the treatment of the family group essential, both to favor the environmental modifications of the group in which the disease originated, to determine the role of each one and to help the family to understand the affected member, accept him and accompany him in his evolution and detect early relapses.

At the beginning of the treatment, it will also be necessary to help the group to cope with the feelings of anger or frustration that patients with an eating disorder provoke in their partners. Also, helping them to understand the phenomenon of the disease by abandoning the feeling that the disorder is voluntary.

Regarding pharmacology, in these cases, it occupies a clearly secondary place. Of course, there is no specific medication for this kind of disorder. Medication may improve some accompanying symptoms or even support it. Few drugs have been approved by the FDA for the treatment of various eating disorders. Among the drugs that have been tried, olanzapine has proven to be of some use in the case of anorexia nervosa, also fluoxetine in binge-eating disorders but without much evidence in bulimia nervosa. However, an adequate psychiatric diagnosis is necessary for the detection and treatment of possible comorbidities that frequently accompany these types of problems.

Pediatric Aspects

Eating behavior disorders are characterized by being patterns anchored in behavior that directly impact physical health. The organic compromise will be reflected in the intake of nutrients with the consequent malnutrition, as well as in the presence of purgative habits.

In anorexia nervosa, the clinical compromise can be flowery in its presentation, according to the level of malnutrition. In contrast, bulimia nervosa can go unnoticed on the physical examination of the clinician, since it does not usually compromise the weight status. In both entities, the organic impact must be sought in the physical examination, as well as in the complementary examinations.

In anamnesis, patients with eating disorders usually report good mood, without asthenia and without pain. The absence of symptoms and the alteration in the body image mark the lack of awareness of the disease and this often makes the therapeutic approach difficult. These patients usually go to the consultation accompanied by a family member and the clinical alarm originates late in the family or in an external institution such as the school.

In younger children, only refusal to ingest and social and emotional withdrawal are usually observed. Sometimes, refusal to eat is usually associated with dehydration, symptoms that require hospitalization.

In older patients, targeted questioning describes a feeling of fullness and chronic constipation resulting from gastroparesis, slowed bowel motility, and poor food intake. Cold intolerance due to loss of subcutaneous cellular tissue is also common. In women, amenorrhea marks a long time of evolution. In men, the decrease in testosterone is more difficult to evidence.

It is important to look for added signs of self-injury such as shallow cut scars on the forearms and hips. Also, it is crucial to bear in mind the reasons that require the hospitalization of our patients: weight loss greater than 30% of the expected weight, extreme bradycardia, arterial hypotension, presence of dehydration, psychiatric risk, lack of family support or intense refusal to eat.

Our Team – Our History

Children's General Hospital Ricardo Gutiérrez was founded in 1875, being the first pediatric hospital in Argentina and in Latin America. It serves the population of children and adolescents from 0 to 18 years old and it is a reference center for the entire country and for Latin America. It is a consulting place for complex pathologies which require the intervention of different pediatric specialties or which cannot be treated in places closer to the patients' home.

Since the middle of the 20th century our hospital has taken in patients with mental health disorders. General Hospital Ricardo Gutiérrez and the Mental Health Unit were pioneers in the hospitalization of mental health patients in a general hospital, always emphasizing the importance of placing them in wards with other different pathologies following an interdisciplinary and comprehensive health conception.

Throughout all these years, this model has been implemented in various ways and has been modified and made more complex, in relation to the characteristics of the patients we have received. The present model of interdisciplinary care for patients with psychic pathologies admitted to the pediatric ward is the product of a long joint work with pediatricians and other specialists of different disciplines.

As it has been mentioned, its origins go back to the beginnings of the 20th century, when the identification of mental problems gradually began, naming them as "the care of nervous diseases." In 1933, a neurology and endocrinology and psychiatry room was put into operation by Dr. Garecio, and later it was led by Dr. Florencio Escardó; who was a pioneer pediatrician in the inclusion of the emotional aspects of childhood pathologies in pediatric training and care. Some of the professionals in this room, influenced by the readings and teachings of Freud and other psychoanalytic masters, developed a way of thinking and understanding pediatric pathology with an integral vision, much more comprehensive than that offered by pediatrics of the time. Dr. Arnaldo Rascovsky, one of the fathers of psychoanalysis in Argentina and Latin America was among them; both he and other colleagues began to observe the symptoms of children from another perspective, deepening the study of somatic manifestations of unconscious conflicts. The close link between pediatrics and psychiatry in the hospital has been deepened, enriched and modified according to the advances of the medical and humanistic sciences, until today.

In Unit 5, a general pediatric hospitalization room, a differentiated sector of four beds was established in 1984 for the hospitalization of adolescent patients, given the specific care in that age group. The patients who were hospitalized for mental health problems were mostly adolescents and these beds were used mainly for the care of eating disorders and, less frequently, psychotic episodes and suicide attempts.

The therapeutic model has been conceived from the very beginning in the antipodes of that which places the mentally ill patient in a place of seclusion and isolation. The patient is hospitalized and remains surrounded by other patients, suffering for different reasons. Thus it is possible to advance towards the demystification of madness, the patient is connoted in a different way, he is a patient like the one who suffers organically or the one who can die. The hospital is then conceived as a space of containment, in a permissive environment for physical and psychological pain.

Our current approach to these patients is carried out by a multidisciplinary team that includes, psychiatrists, psychologists, music therapists, pediatricians, social workers and any other medical specialties that, if necessary, assist our patients. We daily provide each patient with psychiatric treatment, individual, family and group psychotherapy as well as clinical assistance.

The treatments we offer in psychotherapy are all based on psychoanalytic theories, including the group and family therapy. We work in the creation of bonds with other patients. The patient's experience at the hospital allows them to interact and sometimes confront others in a therapeutic environment. Throughout these years we have seen approximately 80 patients per year using this model.

Clinical Report

The case of a child admitted to the hospital will be presented to illustrate the model mentioned above.[1]

Nelson, 11 years old, was hospitalized for presenting symptoms of food restriction with organic risk. He manifested pain in the upper and lower limbs that migrated throughout the evolution of the condition and from the beginning it was addressed jointly with our service.

Due to his initial clinical presentation, the youngster required the intervention of clinical physicians to regain weight and for the treatment of his severe pain. In our area, following our idea of a multiple treatment, he had individual treatment that included psychotherapy, a psychiatrist, and had also family therapy. Besides, he was gradually incorporated into our different group therapies.

In the first encounters with Nelson, he was totally withdrawn, listless, saying he was in pain. During medical check-ups, he frequently asked, "Why do I have to feel so much pain?" This situation generated a certain feeling of desolation and despair within our team, because any attempt to create a better communication was strictly rejected by him. He spent most of the time with therapeutic companions because his mother, the only adult in charge, said that she had to take care of the patient's siblings (all minors), among which there was a little baby.

Regarding his family history, Nelson lived together with his mother and his siblings in a suburban neighborhood, in a house that they shared with other families. Being the sole caregiver of the home, his mother spent much of Nelson's first years doing jobs in which she had to spend long hours (nights included) outside her home.

Nelson and his siblings were left alone or in the care of relatives and suffered various abuses. His father had left them and had not been present at any time during upbringing. His mother said that Nelson's symptoms had begun after the birth of her brother. She explained that they had originated with the aforementioned pains, and that later he began to stop eating. Nelson showed great irritation at the cries of her little child and, at the same time, he demanded that her mother stopped working "so as not to leave the baby alone." In this family, the children appeared as "mouths to feed," with little availability or possibility of differentiating the emotional needs of the different members.

In this first period of hospitalization, Nelson only maintained closer contact with his pediatrician, with whom he began to "negotiate" the repositioning of the nasogastric tube, in exchange for leaving the room.

In the psychotherapy sessions Nelson rejected every therapist's attempt to establish a bond. He transmitted an extreme vulnerability and at the same time he always started shouting and insulting when the therapist appeared. As the days passed, the methods of rejection became more sophisticated, going from "Go away! I don't feel like talking," to singing rap songs full of insults in a very loud voice. The demand was again and again on the side of the therapist. The question was how to find a way in which this attitude could change.

One day, after being expelled once again at Nelson's shouting "Psychologists ask stupid questions!" the therapist suggested that Nelson could be the one to ask the questions. It was then that he asked if he could leave the room. This intervention gave way to a new set of encounters.

They consisted in long walks around the hospital with the previously established rule of not saying a single word. An extremely difficult task for the progress of the therapeutic relationship. Each approach with Nelson had to be carried out with extreme care, any proposal could be read as a demand or as an excessive or abusive demand, causing an immediate withdrawal or strong shows of anger: "You want to make me speak things that I don't want"; "You force me to be here, but I want to go home"; "You cheated on me! I asked you for the computer to look up this information, not to share anything with you!"

We understood these moments of negative transference and of difficulties in accepting help as related to his early experience of lack of care and violence, which generated intense mistrust and anger that were transferred massively to the therapeutic bond. In this way, Nelson was able to dramatize his pain and, by doing so, it began to lessen.

As the patient started to feel less pain, he was able to move and started to go to group therapy and to the different workshops with other patients. As he did so, he started to relate with others, show his own tastes such as rap music and even to establish a romantic relationship with another patient. During a group session, a patient made a comment to Nelson regarding some careless attitude he had had. He immediately reacted aggressively telling the other patient to kill herself. The girl, who had had a suicide attempt, told Nelson that his words really had hurt and had made her feel too much pain. With the help of the group therapists and the comments of other patients, Nelson could realize the painful effect words can have. This issue was later addressed also in his individual therapy.

In family therapy, the first encounters were very difficult to be carried out. Nelson's mother did not want to attend and when she did her words felt very aggressive towards Nelson, we could say they caused pain and they were difficult to be heard even by the family therapists. In later sessions, Nelson was able to manifest his disagreement with his mother and to ask her to bring him different things. In this way he could see if she was there for him and to confirm that some of his demands could be satisfied. His siblings also participated on some occasions, showing much anguish. Two of them were referred to individual therapy. During the sessions, Nelson always made a point that he did not suffer from anorexia and that he had stopped eating because he felt so much pain.

How do we think and understand a case with this interdisciplinary device which uses psychoanalytic theory?

The patients were treated by different psychotherapists, psychiatrists, pediatricians in individual, group and family treatments. All the professionals that worked in these cases meet regularly to think about them together in clinical meetings or supervision sessions to evaluate the progress made and the challenges we have to face.

This 11-year-old boy came with intense pain and suffering. His family, especially his mother, presented several difficulties and had faced many adverse situations. Being a boy who is going through the changes caused by development within this type of family organization was not easy because male figures leave or abandon their wife and children.

How can he accept his body with the changes that it is undergoing? How to feed him when there are many other children to be fed and money is scarce? In our understanding, our patient found it hard to introject or accept the changes in his body and its causes, along with the refusal to eat, a halt in his development and a regression to a former functioning with an acute anguish which translates into somatic pain, which, in turn, triggers a challenge or crossroads (Jeammet, 1994).

Given the transferences we observed in the different therapeutic spaces, we proposed during the admission that the pediatrician should be supportive and should build for the patient the idea of being hosted in a therapeutic space so the patient had the possibility to unfold his conflict and suffering facilitating the start of a psychotherapeutic relationship. This is how anger, rage and anguish surface in the different individual and family consultations but as they are interpreted - the pain in the face of the father's absence, the grieving of a new pregnancy and the birth of a sibling- they stop being physical pain and turn into mental pain and then into an emotion that can be expressed through words.

Note

1 The professionals who treated the patient were Psic. Camila Serra Moledo, Psic. Magdalena Perea, and Dr. Noelia Carranza.

References

Jeammet, P. 1994. El Abordaje psicoanalitico de los trastornos de la conducta alimentaria. *Revista de Psicoanalisis de Niños y Adolescentes* 5.

Kestemberg, J. 1976. *El hambre y el cuerpo*. Espasa Calpe.

Minuchin, S. 1978. *Psychosomatic families: Anorexia nervosa and bulimia nervosa*. Harvard University Press.

Mitchison, D. 2014. The epidemiology of eating disorders Genetic environmental and social factors. *Clinical Epidemiology* 6: 89–97.

Recalcatti, M. 2011. *La última cena: anorexia y bulimia*. Ediciones del cifrado.

Chapter 7

Psychoanalysis and Psycho-oncology
How Each Specialty Enriches the Other

Norman Straker

My psychoanalytic training has allowed me to reach well beyond the couch and provided me with the tools to have an academic career in psycho-oncology, the treatment of cancer patients and their families. My knowledge in psychoanalysis permitted me to introduce basic psychodynamic concepts to the psychiatrists and psychologists on the cancer ward. Similarly, my experience as a psycho-oncologist gave me the opportunity to introduce psychoanalysts to treating cancer patients, dying patients, and patients in grief. The experience of treating patients facing death made me aware of "death anxiety," a neglected concept in psychoanalysis. My understanding of death anxiety as existential issue, has enriched my psychoanalytic practice, teaching and writing.

My journey began as recent graduate of NYPSI in 1976 when I joined the psychiatric service at Sloan Kettering Cancer Center. My psychoanalytic training was key to my being accepted as a voluntary member of the first psychiatric service in a cancer hospital. As the only psychoanalyst I was in a unique position to work with the six full time faculty to develop a modified psychoanalytic psychotherapy to suit the particular challenges of cancer patients. Initially, I led a psychotherapy seminar for the faculty, in which we discussed our approach to the psychotherapy of cancer patients. We read the few psychoanalytic papers on the treatment of patients with cancer (Norton, 1963; Eissler, 1955) that existed and coached each other. In time we began to accept fellows for training, did research, published papers, wrote a book, (Massie, Holland & Straker, 1989) and eventually a fellowship in "psycho-oncology" was established all under the brilliant leadership of Dr. Jimmie Holland.

In the early period of our development and before we were readily consulted for our expertise, our psychiatric service relied on a consultation liaison model to interest oncologists in recognizing the psychological needs of their patients and the need for a referral. The psychiatrists were assigned to various hospital wards and chaired case conferences termed "mental health rounds." My attempts to encourage oncologists to attend these case conferences on the psychosocial issues of their patients was for naught. They

DOI: 10.4324/9781003167679-8

rarely ever joined the nurses, and social workers to discuss their patients, avoiding the realities of the impact of cancer on the lives of their patients and their families.

My psychoanalytic education saw this as a resistance, a defense against a more personal involvement with their sick patients. I was somewhat familiar with that experience, having been a medical doctor before my psychoanalytic training. As an intern and medical student, the person of the patient was an object of study, a person with signs and symptoms that were to be figured out and treated. The experience of working on a cadaver on the first day of medical school was the initial model of the patient–doctor relationship, a dehumanizing object of study. While I had come to medical school with the hope of helping people, my experience after years of grueling study and extremely long hours in the hospital was to become less interested in helping the patient and more interested in doing a good job and surviving. I retrieved my empathy for sick patients during my psychoanalysis and refound my compassion and interest in people.

I was challenged to figure out a method to counter the defense of dehumanizing the patient and treating only the disease. My challenge was to connect the oncologist to their patient as a person. I reasoned that, perhaps if the oncologist could identify himself as a cancer patient, it might allow for a connection, by identification. When I met a movie producer who had recently lost her spouse to cancer, she liked my idea and we agreed to make a film together about doctors with cancer. She had a need to memorialize her husband and I had an interest in seeing if we could reawaken the doctor's empathy through identification. In the movie I interviewed six doctors who were at various stages of their own cancer treatment, or who had recently lost family members to cancer. In the movie *On the Edge of Being: When Doctors Confront Cancer* (Straker & Drazen, 1990) the doctors spoke about the overwhelming importance of feeling cared for, by their doctors as people. They also spoke about their suffering and grief. The movie moved doctors, and medical students who viewed the film. The experience of seeing a colleague with cancer reminded them that "it could be me, and how would I want to be treated."

This film was to become an important teaching devise in medical schools, residency training programs, and a requirement for palliative care doctors. It was translated into Spanish, and Japanese and was shown in Europe and Australia. It was also shown on PBS. I frequently showed the film to oncologists and psychiatrists at medical grand rounds in many cities in the US and Europe. After viewing the film oncologists often spoke publicly for the first time about unresolved feelings, they had about some of the patients. It is important to remember that it was also not considered professional for doctors to have feelings about their patients before the year 2000.

As I noted in my introduction, my analytic training allowed me to work with the faculty in discovering psychotherapeutic interventions for cancer patients. When our fellows arrived, I was invited to lead a twice a week seminar on psychotherapy for more than two decades. Over time I recognized and wrote about certain psychodynamic principles that applied to the understanding of the psychological responses of patients to having cancer and could be helpful in developing basic therapeutic interventions (Straker & Wyszynski, 1986; Straker, 1998, 2008, 2011, 2013, 2019, 2020). I suggested that the patient's psychological response to cancer would be based on the patient's past history, defenses, character, level of attachment and history of coping with adversity. I also suggested that a positive transference would be an extremely valuable therapeutic tool as patients with cancer are very vulnerable and looking for an omnipotent transference rescuer. I further suggested that interventions be directed to establish mastery and bolster usual defenses.

The existence of counter-transferences in all of us who treat cancer patients was a particularly difficult concept for the faculty to accept. They initially believed that any emotional reaction to the patient, their illness, or their suffering was an indication of the therapist's neurosis. In fact, a paper I prepared for presentation for psychiatry grand rounds, to demonstrate common counter-transference reactions, based on some of our psychotherapy cases, was cancelled because the faculty worried, they might be identified as a group of neurotics. It took years of supervision and case conferences for the staff and fellows to share their emotional reactions. Grieving, sadness, anxiety, depression and hypochondriasis are all common in mental health professionals who treat cancer patients. I was pleased when the faculty finally agreed to established counter-transference rounds, as a support for the fellows and encouraged the fellows to have individual therapy.

After we gained sub-specialty status and the department developed a mostly full-time faculty, with a greater integration with the cancer hospital, my teaching role was cut back to supervision, occasional case conferences and four lectures a year on psychoanalytic psychotherapy. This occurred because of the increasing demand for psychiatric consultations from the other departments. Crisis intervention, psycho-pharmacology with supportive psychotherapy, and manualized treatments for dying patients had become the standard of care. This change resulted in limited time for long term individual psychotherapy cases. My lectures were updated to focus on basic psychodynamic principles that applied to all patients regardless of the primary treatment chosen. My new message was that all patients had a transference, defenses, an unconscious, a prior history, and every therapist would have a counter-transference to his patient. Some fellows continued to elect to see patients in individual dynamic therapy but the demand for service limited the available time.

The success and fun I derived from my first movie motivated a second film that focused on an aspect of neglect in the cancer field, the plight and lack of attention, by medical professionals to the spouse of terminally ill patients. A former patient of mine who had lost his wife to pancreatic cancer had a wish to memorialize his wife. After he completed his grief work, and his treatment with me was about to terminate, he began a book project dedicated to his wife. Once completed he decided to present his work to medical audiences to publicize the sale of his book. During his first presentation to the psychiatric department at Sloan Kettering, he choked up and began to grieve, despite the fact that five years had passed since he had lost his wife. I was asked to accompany him for this same lecture to the Sloan Kettering Medical Grand Rounds, based on the upset he had in the prior presentation. I met with him prior to this event. I recommended we film his lecture so he would not have to re- experience his grief with every presentation. He agreed.

After editing the film, I suggested that we could also add a review of his psychotherapy, on film and expose oncologists to the mental health issues of the spouse and illustrate the value of psychotherapy. The film we produced, *The Courage to Survive: Facing the Loss of Your Soulmate* (Straker, 2005) reviewed the challenges faced by the spouse of a terminally ill patient and documented his grief work after she died. He reviewed the highlights of his psychotherapy as an example of treatment that was available to the spouse of a terminally ill cancer patient.

My psychoanalytic training and my treatment of patients with cancer also enriched my psychoanalytic practice. It opened my eyes to a neglected area in psychoanalytic theory and practice. I observed that psychoanalysts generally avoid their analysand's concerns about their mortality, even when they are very sick or dying. Viewing psychoanalysis from the vantage point of a psycho-oncologist I have often marveled at how little interest psychoanalysts seem to have in the role of illness and death.

My survey of articles on psychoanalytic electronic publishing reveals very few recent articles about the treatment of analytic patients with cancer. Three case reports in the classic psychoanalytic journals recommend that an orthodox technique is consistent with the treatment of patients with cancer (Mayer, 1994; McDougal, 2004; Minerbo, 1998). In none of the above reports is the imminence of death and its meaning to the patient discussed in their descriptions of their treatment. In fact, in one of the reports the analysis was "successfully" terminated two weeks before the patient died. These analyses are focused on resolving issues from childhood, while cancer and the patient's looming mortality are neglected. Other journals offer case reports that advocate a modification of technique, especially if the patient is in the advanced stages of illness (Bustamante, 2001). Others suggested that psychotherapy with a dying patient may call for abandoning neutrality, for bending the analytic frame, for facing one's own mortality, and for tolerating the chaotic and unpredictable nature of the course of an illness (Berzoff, 2004). Adams Silvan describes a thoughtful supportive psychoanalytic treatment that is initially modified to help a patient find the strength to fight her terminal illness for two years until she decided to take her own life (Straker, 2013).

As I noted above, the avoidance and denial of death was not limited to the in psychoanalytic literature, it has been my experience as a practicing psychoanalyst to find myself as one of the few psychoanalysts treating cancer patients. I began a Discussion Group at the American Psychoanalytic Meetings on "The Psychoanalytic Psychotherapy and Psychoanalysis of Patients with Cancer," more than 35 years ago, which continues to this day. The attendance at these early meeting rarely exceeded five to ten participants. However, the numbers began to increase as the treatments for cancer improved. Now patients in analysis who develop cancer are staying in analysis rather than terminating, as in the past. Also, patients who developed cancer are now more anxious for psychiatric treatments. In the last decade a critical mass of thirty-five to forty psychoanalysts attended these meetings.

The vast majority of analysts who chose to present their cases do so, because their cases had stalled, nothing new was happening. Repeatedly, the problem was that neither the patient nor the analyst would bring up the patient's concerns about dying (the elephant in the room). Death anxiety usually triggers counter-transference reactions such as anxiety, identification and impotence in the analyst. Avoidance or a collusion with the patient's denial is the result and the case is stalled. The reluctance of psychoanalysts to venture into this uncomfortable territory without a road map is obvious. The patients pick up on this and collude with their analyst to leave death out of the sessions, despite its being the major concern of the patient. Therefore, no progress in the treatment is made.

Why have we analysts been reluctant to raise the issues of mortality with our patients and participate in their existential challenge? This is because "death anxiety" and its unconscious defenses are poorly understood by psychoanalysts. Freud's theories which described death anxiety as a derivative of the anxieties of childhood is of little help when working with patients or in supervision. The therapist's linking the patient's current life crisis of facing death with the anxieties of childhood is insufficient to help the patient master their circumstances. The flood of feelings unleashed when facing death of anguish, sadness, grief, and terror are not ameliorated or lessened when the therapists link the present with past anxieties. This intervention is totally ineffective and does not bring about any solace. This state of affairs is very unsatisfactory and feels unempathic. I struggled for decades with trying to find a solution to it.

My search for a solution led me to pursue an understanding of death anxiety from existential psychoanalysis and empirical data about the unconscious defenses against death anxiety. I turned my attention to existential psychoanalysis, Irvin Yalom and Ernst Becker to get a better understanding of death anxiety. Becker wrote his Pulitzer Prize-winning book *The Denial of Death* in 1973. Contrary to Freud, Becker believed that all human activity is largely driven by unconscious efforts to deny and transcend death. He hypothesized that we build character and culture to shield ourselves from the devastating awareness of our underlying helplessness and terror of our inevitable death (Becker, 1973). Yalom describes death transcendence as a major motif in all our defenses, dreams, monuments, theology, ideology, drive to get ahead, yearning for lasting fame, and drive for symbolic immortality (Yalom, 1980).

Sheldon Solomon undertook the task of empirically validating Becker's hypothesis. He designed research studies that demonstrated the existence of unconscious death anxiety and its defenses, known as "terror management theory" (Solomon et al., 1998, 2015). The main tenets of terror management theory are: As long as we are valuable members of our culture and we achieve a feeling of personal significance and high self-esteem we create a path to symbolic immortality and lessen our fear of death. Similarly, sustaining faith in our cultural worldview offers us order, meaning, and permanence and lessens our death anxiety.

William Breitbart's research on the importance of terminally ill patients finding meaning in their suffering demonstrated that a focus on meaning in therapy improves spiritual well-being and lessens anxiety, demoralization, and a desire for death. His research was based on Viktor Frankl's logotherapy (Breitbart et al., 2010; Frankl, 1963). A variation of this same theme emerged in the palliative care literature and was termed "whole person care" (Hutchinson, 2011). It aims for healing. Healing comes from the acceptance that cure is no longer possible and a redirecting of the patient to achievable hopes and goals. It is believed to occur through a healing connection from caring caretakers (Mount & Boston, 2007).

Solomon and Breitbart's research findings and the recommendations of "whole person medicine" convinced me that psychological interventions based on these findings should be added to my psychoanalytic psychotherapy for patients facing death as a means to bring solace, and healing to the patient and a sense of competence to the therapist. Effective therapeutic interventions make avoidance and denial unnecessary. The experimental demonstration that death anxiety is lessened by contributing to one's community and having high self-esteem, provides a strong rationale for recommending that therapists validate their dying patient's life achievements. As patients tells their life story, the therapist should acknowledge the value of patient's work and role in the family and community. For example, if the patient was a teacher, expressing admiration for their contribution to many young people they taught is suggested. Similarly, if the patient was a doctor, a review of the many important diagnoses that saved lives might be discussed. If the patient has children or grandchildren, an exploration of their lives, and futures as well as the patient's relationship in their formative years increases self-esteem. A focus on all or any of the patient's contributions, especially those that will live on beyond their life span, can contribute to sense of symbolic immortality and the view that their life had value and meaning. If your patient is a young mother, with terminal cancer who is despondent that her children will lose their mother, you as the therapist can try to help her "go on mothering." I have made the following suggestions to some of my patients; she can train a caregiver to bring up her children with her values, she can write letters or make videotapes with messages that can be opened or viewed on special occasions as per example; when the child is ready for college gets engaged. Finally, an exploration of the patient's religious views, especially in regards, to a belief in an after -life, or reunion fantasies with parents or lost love ones is often very comforting.

Despondency, with a desire for death, is a problematic state of mind and has not been shown to respond to antidepressants (Breitbart et al., 2000). It can be best be managed by focusing on finding meaning with the patient in the present and pursuing important goals that can be met. This might include encouraging a greater engagement with friends and family, helping one's children feel valued, focusing on healing relationships that have become frayed, facing regrets, and finally a focus on spirituality.

Case Study

Phil (not his real name) was a very energetic 80-year-old married man who looked much younger than his age. Phil was referred to me with a diagnosis of pancreatic cancer and a 3- to 6-month prognosis. He was receiving chemotherapy and opiates for pain, when I first met him. His chief complaints were panic attacks and a deep depression. He was counting down the days until he was expected to die and preparing for his death. He was arranging a goodbye party for himself. He had also compiled a list of speakers for his memorial service and had visited the chapel where his memorial service would be held. He was mostly concerned about the future of his two adult daughters and his wife.

Phil had lived the American Dream. His parents were from eastern Europe. He was born and raised in the Bronx. He worked his way through college, and he became a successful Wall Street money manager. He married a woman whom he described as "a beauty." They were very social in New York. They lived in a large West Side apartment and owned a home in Greenwich, Connecticut. Phil considered himself an intellectual and was very vocal about current affairs. He was very philanthropic, wrote many letters to the editor of the *New York Times*, had a blog with many followers and also had many friends in Israel.

In my first meeting he did not appear to me like a dying person with only 3 to 6 months to live. His good color and his robust presentation were impressive given his prognosis. He was anxious and spoke about his imminent death with sadness. He was depressed but wanted to live as long as he could. He spoke about his life, his acquaintances, and his writings with great pride. He and his wife had been a dashing couple and socialized with the rich and famous.

My initial comments were that I was most impressed with how well he looked and that I had seen many patients before with pancreatic cancer and he was in no way typical. I did not believe he was dying imminently and suggested that rather than a good-bye party, which I believed to be premature, he might consider a party to celebrate his remarkable life. I also recommended he try to drop the 3- to 6-month prognosis and try to "live with uncertainty." I said we would both know when he was weak and near the end, but it certainly did not seem imminent to me.

We agreed on a once-weekly psychotherapy, which he very much enjoyed. I prescribed fluoxetine up to 40 mg with clonazepam 0.5 mg twice a day and clonazepam 0.125 mg wafers for panic attacks and a depressive disorder. I began each session remarking on his healthy physical appearance, which lasted up until two weeks before he died. This was a very important intervention, as it was reassuring to a man who had been told he was going to die imminently. His panic attacks decreased in response to the meds, the acceptance of living with uncertainty, his busy schedule, and our psychotherapy. We spent the majority of time talking about the testimonials he was receiving from emails from around the world and his many important visitors. Clearly, these activities fueled his unconscious defenses against death anxiety. I routinely reinforced these defenses by validating his contributions to his community and noting the important people who were eager to seek his counsel and meet with him. It was important for him to know that he would not be forgotten and that his contributions would live on indefinitely. He was also very proud of his daughters and grandchildren. He was troubled that he would not be available to take care of them as he always had. He reviewed his marriage with great fondness and joyously recalled the trips he and his wife had taken together.

Aside from his presenting symptoms, Phil was interested in my admiring him as a special person, suggesting a narcissistic personality disorder. It seemed important to him that I appreciate his life achievements. At the same time, Phil seemed to respect my expertise and desire to help him. Aside from whatever positive transference there was, it was also an authentic relationship of mutual respect. In fact, other than his relationship with me, he was quite alienated. He could not confide in his wife, who was depressed and tearful, and he could not confide in his daughters or grandchildren.

After about six months, we began to address the issue that most distressed him. He had failed to sell his firm's stock before it went bankrupt. The majority of the family's assets had been held in this company. He had felt stupid and could not forgive himself for being in denial about the seriousness of the financial crisis. My repeated offering was that few people had anticipated the severity of the crisis and its rapidity. Many people were frozen as stocks tumbled precipitously. I had other bankers as patients, and they had all suffered serious losses. Over time, I think he was able to forgive himself. I also reminded him that there would still be significant resources left after he passed and that his children were well educated, well traveled, and exposed to the finer things in life.

As I mentioned earlier, Phil had been well until two weeks before he died. He cancelled his last two appointments because he wasn't feeling up to coming to my office. He declined my request to make a home visit. I suspect he did not want me to see him sick. He was very proud of his appearance. I was informed by one of his daughters that he died exactly one year after our first visit. I was very saddened but took some comfort from the fact that he had really "lived" the last eleven months and he had accepted the idea that he was no less negligent than everyone else regarding the stock market crash.

This brief case summary illustrates the importance of not accepting imminent death, living with uncertainty, focusing on celebrating a life well lived, reconnecting with old friends and acquaintances, accepting testimonials, saying goodbye, and forgiving oneself for one's imperfections. After his panic had dissipated and he had stopped thinking about how little time he had, the sessions for the most part were joyful, and he took great pride in recounting to me his life's journey, the important people he knew, and the many people who wanted to reconnect with him. I believe my validation of his life was helpful in diminishing his death anxiety and panic. The relationship was real and meaningful, as I was the only person he really talked with – although it was somewhat puzzling, that he did not say good-bye to me. The medications played an important role as well.

These two major interventions, which are evidenced based help the psychoanalyst work with patients facing death with a sense of competence and a belief that they can be with their patient in a meaningful way. This is in sharp contrast to avoidance and denial, which had been the most common reactions of psychoanalysts in the past. It is also a far more empathic and meaningful approach than a cognitive therapy designed to make death less frightening (if that is even possible).

References

Becker, E. (1973). *The denial of death*. New York: Free Press.
Berzoff, J. (2004). When a client dies: A commentary. *Psychoanalytic Social Work*, 11.
Breitbart, W., Rosenfeld, B., Gibson C., *et al.* (2010). Meaning-centered group psychotherapy for patients with advanced cancer: A pilot randomized control study. *Psycho-oncology*, 19, 21–28.
Breitbart, W., Rosenfeld, B., Pessin, H., Kim, M., Funesti-Esch, J., Galietta, M., Nelson, C. J. & Bresci, R. (2000). Depression, hopelessness, and desire for hastened death in terminally ill patients with cancer. *Journal of the American Medical Association*, 284, 2907–2911.
Bustamante, J. J. (2001). Understanding hope: Persons in the process of dying. *International Forum of Psychoanalysis*, 10(1), 49–55.
Eissler, K. (1955) *The dying patient*. New York: International University Press.
Frankl, V. (1963). *Man's search for meaning*. Boston, MA: Beacon Press.

Massie, M. J., Holland, J. C. & Straker, N. (1989). Psychotherapeutic interventions. In J. C. Holland & J. H. Rowland (Eds.), *Handbook of Psycho-oncology: Psychological care of the patient with cancer* (pp.). New York: Oxford University Press.

Mayer, E. I. (1994). Some implications for psychoanalytic technique drawn from the analysis of a dying patient. *Psychoanalytic Quarterly*, 63, 1.

McDougal, J. (2004). The psychoanalytic voyage of a breast-cancer patient. *The Annual of Psychoanalysis*, 32, 9–28.

Minerbo, V. (1998). The patient without a couch: An analysis of a patient with terminal cancer. *International Journal of Psychoanalysis*, 79, 83.

Mount, B. F. & Boston, P. H. (2007). Healing connections: On moving from suffering to a sense of well-being. *Journal of Pain Symptom Management*, 33(4), 372–388.

Norton, J. (1963). The treatment of a dying patient. *Psychoanalytic Study of the Child*, 18(1), 540–560.

Solomon, S., Greenberg, J. & Pyszynsi, T., (1998). Tales from the crypt: On the role of death in life. *Zygon*, 33(1), 9–43.

Solomon, S., Greenberg, J. & Pyszczynski T. (2015). *The worm at the core: On the role of death in life*. New York: Random House.

Straker, N. (1998). Psychodynamic psychotherapy for cancer patients. *Journal of Psychotherapy Practice and Research*, 7, 11–19.

Straker, N. (2005). The courage to survive: Facing the loss of your soulmate. Video presentation. Retrieved from www.internationalpsychoanalysis.net.

Straker, N. (2008). Dynamic psychotherapy for cancer patients and their spouses. *Psychiatric Times*, 8(9), 119–121.

Straker, N. (2011). The courage to survive: Facing the loss of your soulmate. *Palliative and Supportive Care*, 9, 2.

Straker, N. (2013). *Facing cancer and the fear of death: A psychoanalytic perspective on treatment*. Lanham, MD: Rowman & Littlefield.

Straker, N. (2019). Psychodynamic psychotherapy for patients with cancer, survivorship. *Journal of Psychodynamic Psychiatry*, 47(4), 403–424.

Straker, N. (2020). The treatment of patients who die. *Journal of Psychodynamic Psychiatry*, 48(1), 1–25.

Straker, N. & Drazen, R. (1990). On the edge of being: When doctors confront cancer. Video presentation. Retrieved from www.internationalpsychoanalysis.net.

Straker, N. & Wyszynski, A. (1986). Denial in the cancer patient: A common-sense approach. *International Medicine for the Specialist*, 7, 150–155.

Yalom, I. (1980). *Existential psychotherapy*. New York: Basic Books.

Chapter 8

Psychodynamic Contributions to Palliative Care Patients and their Family Members

Linda Emanuel

Introduction

Recently, a parent of lower and middle school children whose terminally ill spouse had been told that little time was left said: "I don't know how to talk with the kids about this; they don't get it and I don't get what's happening either." I responded, as I often do, with something like: "It helps many to think together about what death means; it helps children and adults alike to explore; agreement doesn't matter so much. It sounds simple, silly almost, but it seems to improve many things if people have a way of thinking about death.'

Indeed, this may seem like an odd thing to say to the reader too. Freud asserted that death is not represented in the unconscious and that it is not possible for an existing entity to conceptualize non-existence (Freud, 1915). Yet, something is necessary and possible; we can and often do represent death in our minds and doing so or not seems to make a big difference (De Masi, 2004).

Indeed, this distressed parent sighed with what seemed like a bit of relief. The conversation went on, ending with: "One thing that will continue for sure is the love; the kids can understand that. I just worry about the other stuff that will continue – the guilt, the anger – we weren't perfect." "Yes, that's usually so." I said, "But we can address that; kids can find a realistic way of thinking about that too; its human nature and its OK; love is never simple."

This encounter was part of a palliative care-based family-oriented dynamic therapy. In psychoanalytic work, the unit of care is the analysand. In palliative care, it is the (patient-defined) family, and care is designed to start with illness onset and continue through the bereavement journey. As usual, I had worked with members of this family, separately and together. We were midway through a long journey. The transference and countertransference was more complicated than with traditional single-person analyses but still grist for the mill, and not more complicated than being a grandmother or aunt/uncle figure, which is close to how they used me too.

DOI: 10.4324/9781003167679-9

The hospice and palliative medicine discipline is a relatively recent addition to modern medicine (Clark, 2018). It began several decades ago by building on the observation that some people were inspiringly able to find peace and equanimity in their time of dying, while by contrast, others suffered apparently needlessly terribly. It also noted, as Freud had, that the bereaved seemed to have similarly contrasting possible experiences; some were able to grieve the loss of a loved one in what seemed a healthy way while others seemed to be stuck and to suffer interminably (Freud, 1917). The field of hospice and palliative medicine set out to help people to "die well" and to "mourn healthily;" psycho-oncology became a sub-specialty (Holland et al., 1998). This chapter considers how psychodynamic care can contribute through the fostering of existential maturity (Emanuel et al., 2020), a term that roughly designates whatever it takes to have a healthy albeit painful experience of loss, death, and bereavement (Emanuel et al., 2017).

What Is Existential Maturity?

Existential maturity is a capacity to "die well" and/or "mourn healthily." Other terms and descriptions exist. Some refer to an oscillating prognostic awareness, which is probably a description of the same, or getting to the same (Jackson et al., 2013). Others describe existential terror or death anxiety, which are probably the obverse (Solomon et al., 2015; Becker, 1973). The specific term chosen is less important than having terms we can use. A working definition of existential maturity is: the ability to handle mortality without maladaptive defenses that interfere with the work and achievements of the last phase of life. To the extent that adapting to mortality requires processing grief for living that will not happen (Knight & Emanuel, 2007), and bereavement requires remaking the self-structures that the deceased person supported, a way of describing what is involved in existential maturity is: the capacity to grieve what mortality cuts off.

The definition could feel judgmental – a right way to die, a right way to mourn. This would be unfortunate, because psychodynamic and palliative medicine approaches both eschew judgment and imposition of goals. Everyone dies their own way and everyone mourns in their own way. However, both palliative medicine and psychodynamic practices also recognize that people come seeking relief from psychological suffering and damaging states and hoping for vitality, integration, intimacy, and resilience. For some psychoanalysts, the above definition and description of what it entails are far too broad since so much of the work of psychoanalysis turns out to be about grieving. However, that seems acceptable because it may be that existential maturity is very much of a feather with other types of analytic growth and development – simply focused on evolving ways to cope with the stark realities of mortality.

Two further notes belongs here. One is that this chapter discusses existential maturity as an attribute of *a* person. Realistically, it is probably also an attribute of *people* who interact around matters of mortality. Those people may be part of the therapeutic dyad (Emanuel et al., 2017), a spousal couple (Jackson et al., 2013), a family (Ahluwalia et al., 2020), a medical care team (Robert, 2012), a community, or a culture. Future work should explore intersubjective (Atwood & Stolorow, 1984) and group systems perspectives (Petriglieri & Petriglieri, 2020) on existential maturity. However, this chapter focuses on what it is from the individual perspective and on how it develops.

The second note relates to a common assumption that existential maturity comes with age. It might be easier to die old than young; a life cut short misses the potential that a longer life may have realized. However, observation does not suggest a tight link between mature years and existential maturity. An elder who is frantic with fear of dying and a child dying of cancer with serenity and love come readily to mind for people who work with the dying. Pediatric palliative care clinicians universally acknowledge that children can be awe-inspiringly mature in the way they approach their dying. So existential maturity is probably not a straightforwardly Eriksonian kind of last developmental stage (Erikson, 1982). At the same time, people do seem to find their own version of existential maturity in a manner that is life-stage appropriate. For instance, a dying child's drawings or those of a child facing bereavement are not the same as an adult artists' work when facing the same. For instance, a 6-year-old boy whose parent was dying drew a picture of a winding path by a stream with the ill parent way in the distance, very small, in a cave and the other parent foregrounded, running scared off the path with panic on her face. The boy himself was floating off to the side, drawn last. In the other situation, a single artist (who used them/they/their pronouns) in their late 30s was anticipating imminent bereavement. They made artwork about trash and decay. Both the child and the adult were capable of symbolizing death but did so as was relevant for that individual's stage and needs. Humans apparently deal with existential matters from our beginning. People appear to handle this challenge in varied and more or less adaptive ways throughout life. Existential maturity can be thought of as an age-appropriate ability to handle mortality without becoming unmoored.

Two Cases

Case 1

Angela was 48 years old when, having lived with cancer for 5 years, she was coming to the end. She had been raised by a wealthy, demanding grandmother, a rarely available father, and a lonely mother who was deeply invested in but materialistic with her children. The siblings were competitive. Angela, the favored sibling, felt she had been successful in holding the family together across generations by virtue of success in her grandmother-chosen career, attractiveness, and her accomplished husband and children. Angela approached her cancer encounters as competitive events; her metaphors were of winning sports games. When she was beset by symptoms or when treatments failed, she took refuge in entitlement; if one family member declined the special care that held her together, she would feel hurt and turn to another who offered. As Angela's prognosis shortened and illness overtook her days and her body, she felt increasingly like a failure. Any lapse in attentive care and admiration prompted her to inquire about assisted suicide, something that re-garnered the buoying attention. Angela's sessions continued until she was unable to recover from a procedure. She rallied from her barely conscious state long enough to tell her surrounding family that she loved them before passing.

Psychodynamic work had occurred over a period of several years. It was aided by Angela's prior experience of therapy, innate ability, and her desire to be psychologically healthy. She and her family enjoyed many, often playful, quality times. She also tangibly prepared for death, arranging her affairs, writing letters for her children to grow up with and her husband to hold dear, and talking openly about their hopes and fears. However, her physical suffering narrowed her focus, and inevitable absorption with her illness and its treatments took away from being present with her family. Her chemotherapy had affected her memory, her executive functioning, and seemed to impede her relational attunement too. Her family noted that she was more demanding and her considerateness less deft, leaving them feeling like unwilling servants; she in turn felt abandoned. When the family realized they were all defensively responding to the growing separation that the illness and anticipated loss/death made inevitable (Robert, 2012), they felt compassion for one another and managed well again until the next cycle.

Interpretive work was not obviously resisted, being thoughtfully acknowledged, but did not seem to open up new curiosity or growth, something I attributed to not only the usual defenses but to the neurological impact of chemotherapy on her ability to make new meaning and thereby deepen the work. A good deal of time was spent mirroring, which the patient seemed to increasingly dependent on to understand where she was emotionally.

Noticeably, Angela treated me with careful respect; in the countertransference, I felt I could understand how she held herself together by being a successful rendition of her mother and grandmother's aspirations. The security of her attachment to her objects depended on her being a winner. So losing the battle with cancer, and especially when her family left her without the special care that made her feel successful, plunged her into a state that felt worse than death to her. Suggestive interpretations aimed at understanding her main defense (that her success made the world all right) were met with confusion and I judged there was neither time nor sufficient merit in any attempt to re-narrate this core belief. I felt she was more together, more cohesive, less vulnerable to feeling suicidal, when she felt like a success in my eyes for having navigated the dying journey well. It was a struggle to keep the transference deep enough that this version of success kept working, but this was the best holding I could find for her.

Angela was not able to engage the full potential of analytic work, but she was able to use it in her own way. She maintained her cohesion by using the mirroring from our sessions to replace the self-understanding that chemotherapy and her illness seemed to have taken away. She was able to use a more adaptive defense of "dying well" rather than unrealistically beating her terminal illness. Although limited, this holding and partial adaptive coping probably limited the dysregulated emptiness that made her seem demanding to her family and felt desperate for her.

Case 2

At 70, Braun had been diagnosed with cancer a year prior, had completed anti-cancer treatment and was to be maintained on a low dose of chemotherapy. He had few symptoms but he had been told that he had less than an even chance of living three more years. The situation ushered in reflection about how to live his remaining life and how to face mortality. Death, he protested, was simply nothingness so why was he so rattled? Braun had engaged in analysis years before but had ended it when a job caused him to move cities. On learning at the time that "the saying goodbye part of analysis could take many months," he rejected that as ridiculous and ended the analysis rather abruptly. Now he felt that he did not know what saying goodbye well entails and that it might help him face dying.

During our two-year analysis, in which time his cancer did not return, Braun returned to some of his unresolved relationships, both past and present, finding new ways of understanding them and finding compassion and appreciation for people who had previously felt impinging or inadequate. His regrets over finding less success in his career than he'd aspired to faded as he discovered a greater identification in his retirement occupation of portrait sketching, and in being an active grandfather.

However, ending this second analysis with me turned out to be hard and he surprised himself by how he felt incomplete and lost in heaviness, or angry with me, on long weekends and during my vacation. Associating to this sensation, he recalled how absent his mother seemed to him to be when he needed her. In a screen memory, he recalled receiving a bloody head gash at the hands of a rock-throwing fellow second grader on the playground that prompted him to break out of the playground and run home. His mother did not take him to a doctor as he expected, but reprimanded him for leaving school and sent him back. When I said: "It must have felt like your mother was really not there for you … if only she had scooped you up and felt your fright and sought real help for the big gash in your head," his face contorted.

We acknowledged that his mother's deadness to him had travelled with him all the years of his life so far.

This was a mutative moment for Braun. As we worked this new level of understanding through in subsequent sessions, new meaning was created about what frightened Braun most about dying: it was that sensation of mother being not there for him when he was mortally afraid, of emptiness, of not mattering, of being bad for having sought her vital safety. That was his representation of death. Now Braun recreated his conception of and expectations for dying. He understood living as loving connections and understood dying as a succession of connection, not so much the psychic death from his mother's absent care. His focus consolidated around his family and friends; his paintings were for them. His relationships, he felt, were sufficient reason to be peaceful about dying. They, he said, would be his continuity.

A Psychoanalytic Perspective on Meaning-Making about Mortality

Meaning-Making or Symbolization in Serious Illness Settings

Psycho-spiritual perspectives in palliative care literature on the needs of people focus in great part on meaning-making (Mackay and Bluck, 2010; Pargament, 2007; Emanuel et al., 2015; Johnson et al., 2020). Interventions that aid creation of narrative meaning and connection bolster dignity and bring comfort and gratification to the bereaved (Chochinov, 2011; Breitbart et al., 2015). When it comes to making meaning of the ultimate existential matters (What does life mean? What does death mean? Where do meaningful relationships fit in this?), people are often working in their minds at the same level at which psychoanalysis works. Psychoanalytic/dynamic work can measurably and lastingly improve a person's impeded ability to use meaning making in matters of work, love, and play (Shedler, 2010). Therefore, it makes sense that analytic/dynamic work can improve a person's ability to make meaning of existential matters and go about the tasks of dying. Braun and Angela both adjusted their meaning significantly.

Braun realized that his conception of death was actually psychological deadness (De Masi, 2004; Green, 1993). As he grew in understanding about his internalized psychic deadness that came from his emotionally absent mother, he felt more connected to his deceased mother and he grew in his desire and ability to redouble his investments in meaningful relationships. He conceived now of death as being like a fond farewell in which he would stay in the minds of his surviving loved ones. He seemed to lack a narrative (Joe Schwartz, October 2020, verbal communication) for his sensation of absence until the therapeutic relationship allowed him to understand and share what had happened to him in that screen memory incident and on so many other occasions.

Angela was not fully able to adjust her way of thinking about death to something so fulfilling. She still thought of death as a failure. Success was living the life that her mother and grandmother found exemplary. However, Angela was able to see dying well as a substitute form of success and that did help her, even though she remained dependent on those around her for holding her together at each new failure to cure her incurable illness.

Trauma-Like Disruptions

Turning to the question of what is the psychological mechanism by which humans make meaning of mortality, assistance is available from the work of Bion. Traumatized patients characteristically have disruptions in narrative coherence and difficulties with affect regulation – two essential elements of meaning making (Mackay and Bluck, 2010). Observations by Bion with "shell-shocked" veterans of war lead him toward his theory of meaning making (Bion, 1962). His theory, expounded on by many psychoanalytic scholars since, describes the meaning-making equipment that is used in a child's early meaningful relationships and continues through life. Its application below is simplistic but hopefully helpful.

Seen through the lens of Bionian thought, the person grappling with mortality and its associated losses is beset with raw, devastating feelings that do not seem thinkable (Bion called these beta elements; perhaps that was the nothingness that Braun experienced). The palliative care team and perhaps specifically the psychotherapist, the family's care for one another, and interventions such as those cited above all provide interactions in which the person can receive their response to the unthinkable feelings (Bion called this alpha function). The outcome for the person is some way of thinking about it (Bion called these metabolized, symbolized K elements). That is, the person facing mortality arrives at a way of thinking about and understanding death and loss that works for them. They have made meaning; they have symbolized the otherwise unmanageable reality; now they can settle. Maladaptive defenses are not necessary; reality – along with the affect and cognizance that goes with it – is, if undesirable, manageable. Perhaps even the eventual, ultimate ability is the ability to sit with what Bion called "O," or the unknowable of what is death, and allow it.

One way of understanding what happens to disrupt the meaning making that affords existential maturity is similar to the way Bion understood trauma. Bion understood trauma to disrupt the linking between a person's raw unthinkable sensations (beta elements) and the protective figure's meaning-making (alpha) function (Bion, 1961). Perhaps disruptions or non-development of linking regarding mortality also prevent development of existential maturity. The extent of those disruptions might have to do with the "dose" of mortality-salient experience that has too little alpha function. A child or adult with exposure to death and loss with plenty of alpha function may develop meaning and existential maturity (Emanuel, 2020). A person with similar exposure and too little alpha function may be unable to make meaning and become functionally traumatized, unable to develop existential maturity. One clinician recently remarked during case review of an analysis that perhaps existential maturity is the opposite of a traumatized state (Robert Galatzer-Levy, October 2020, verbal communication).

The relationship of Kleinian and Bionian thought, both as applied to the mechanism of existential maturity, commands attention. This is especially so since Kleinian theory entails oscillating between polarized positions and palliative care emphasizes oscillation that allows people facing mortality to reach some kind of understanding within the holding embrace of palliative care (Emanuel et al., 2017). Bionian models entail a to and fro within a relationship as well. The Kleinian infant tussles desperately with existential anxiety and receives (or does not) comfort in the connected, depressive position that allows cradled, connected existence. The Bionian child tussles with meaning making and finds (or does not) metabolized, affectively–conceptually linked understanding in the (alpha) milieu of a nurturing relationship.

Angela can be understood as the Kleinian child who always needed help, and paid heavily, to reach the depressive position. Alternatively, she can be understood as the Bionian child who had difficulty finding and using the relational meaning-making (alpha) function and was often left with unmetabolized (beta) elements and less useable understanding (K elements). She did evolve her way of thinking about death and did make use of the relationships she had, but it was limited. Was she traumatized? Perhaps facing mortality was itself so traumatizing for Angela that it interrupted her adaptive, meaning-making functions. However, it also seemed that her core coping mode (success) and the impact of her chemotherapy on her brain might have been to blame for her inability to make use of interpretation to create new meaning and her newly inept relatedness. Perhaps the effect on the meaning-making and relationship-connecting functions of our human minds is comparable to chronic micro-trauma.

Braun by contrast had made use of his first analysis to create meaningful relatedness from understanding, and brought this capacity to his second analysis and his confrontation with mortality. He evolved his understanding of death and adjusted his self-structure to integrate that new understanding. This was evident in his adapted identity and emphasis on relationships with family members who would survive him; his efforts to create continuity through love and legacy were realistic. In addition, he had a companion in the journey (his analyst) with whom he had a relationship in which there was active acknowledgment of the finitude of his life (Stephany Brody, verbal communication). Perhaps his was the opposite of a traumatic state.

Relationship to Attachment

Palliative medicine clinicians have long noted that people often die the same way they lived. As the adage goes: an angry person dies angry; a fighter fights to the end; an anxious person dies with anxiety; and a loving person dies lovingly. A member of a psychologically minded team of palliative care physicians deepened this observation with her curiosity over the connection between a person's attachment style and the way they die; do people with a secure attachment die more gently, for instance, while people with anxious attachment styles have more fear (Bowlby, 1958; Keri Brenner, 2018, verbal communication)?

An important related possibility emerged during a case review that transference attachment might be a good indicator of existential maturity (Molly Witten, October 2020, verbal communication). Further, the possibility emerged that as a person approaches mortality they seek a unique kind of attachment object: someone to accompany and guide the person "across the River Styx" (Phil Lebovitz, October 2020, verbal communication). Certainly, ancient legends corroborate such a figure's meaning. Whereas the archetypal mother brings the child into the world, an archetypal boatman ushers the exit. Charon the boatman is depicted as a harsh figure, but perhaps that stems from anxiety and perhaps it yields to a nurturing figure as a person finds greater levels of existential maturity. In this way of thinking, and accepting that earlier attachment experiences affect subsequent ones, it makes sense that attachment style would affect a person's ability to use relationships to help face mortality.

It makes intuitive sense that there might be an inherent connection between Bowlby's and Bion's perspectives on a person's subjective reality since attachment style can readily been seen as a reflection of the relationship between the child who brings unprocessed experience (the beta elements) and the parent-figure who brings the processing (alpha function). It may even make sense to think of the psychological mechanism or working apparatus of existential maturity as part of both. For instance, one way of understanding death anxiety is a failure to use the attachment relationship to manage the fear. This is consistent with Kleinian thought; perhaps the death drive is internally directed rage at attachment failure.

The connection between attachment style and meaning making should also alert us to the importance of interpersonal connection in how a person dies and what might constitute a natural process for bolstering existential maturity when families come together around a dying loved one. A consensus statement from a palliative care group interested in psychological aspects of terminal illness noted that strengthening attachments is a notable feature for many patients (Brenner et al., submitted).

Angela had an anxious attachment style. Her dependence on her family and therapist for admiring encouragement and affirmations of success were continuations of her pre-illness relationships and she could become seriously anxious then dark if these relational needs were not met.

Braun by contrast seemed to have a fairly secure attachment style. His family history and pre-analytic style was disorganized, but a good analysis had apparently repaired a good deal for him. He was able to use the therapeutic and family relationships to find meaning and face mortality with a good deal of peaceful love.

Oscillating Positions and Transitional Space

It is not surprising that existential struggles takes us to the core of other major analytic thought as well. Kleinian thought also helps us make sense of existential maturity (Klein, 1935). Solving the crisis of mind that Klein attributed to infants comes up for the dying and bereaved quite intensely. We attribute to the Kleinian infant these crises: Am I part of you, since my existence depends on you? Am I annihilated if I am separated from you? How can you put me down? How can I return to your embrace? Perhaps the dying person recasts the same concerns as questions like: You are part of me, so how do I die and leave you here? Or for the bereaved: Does part of me die as you cease to be there? How can you leave me? How do I become fully me again if you die?

One way of understanding Braun's development is that he had more and more comfort with the depressive position. Angela also sought the depressive position and the conflict entailed in so doing during health was substituted for a more adaptive one, but it remained not entirely her own and was hard to use. She was less individuated and more dependent than was Braun on his loved ones; she was more often in the paranoid schizoid position – times when assisted suicide appealed to her.

Klein hypothesized how infants reach the depressive position. People facing the myriad losses that precede their death and anticipating the ultimate loss of life can tell us more than infants can about how they reach the depressive position. An interesting feature of people bereaved of an "essential other," or a highly important internal object (Galatzer-Levy & Cohler, 1993), is that they often are furious at the person for having died, and at other times often feel guilty that they killed the person.

Angela sustained greater compromise than Braun sustained and she was able to access and share less of her unconscious process. Braun, who had achieved more functional object relations and individuation to the point of being able to take responsibility for his limitations, appeared to reach the depressive position through intimate connections that were purpose designed to last beyond death. However, before he managed this, it seems to have been important that Braun could process his anger at his former analyst for allowing such an abrupt termination and his own guilt at doing so. Perhaps there was also some address of an unconscious Kleinian sense that he killed his former analyst too. He seemed better able to complete his preparation for his mortality after becoming familiar and comfortable with this aggressive aspect of himself (Denia Barrett, October 2020, verbal communication).

Another major psychoanalytic scholar whose work has great relevance for existential maturity is Winnicott. The two major notions for which he is most known are both relevant. First, fragmentation (Winnicott, 1974). It seems that the sensation of falling, of fragmenting, provide good descriptions of the falling apart that happened to Angela when she could not get enough tender care from her family; her thoughts of assisted suicide were to foreshorten and end that feeling. It seems many people who greatly fear death associate that feeling with or believe it to be the same as death (De Masi, 2004).

Winnicott's other foundational idea of transitional space – which we can understand here as the therapeutic or analytic space where there is openness to creativity from the unconscious – is also relevant (Winnicott, 1965). It is in the safe transitional space created by the parent figure that the child explores and creates a manageable and useable relationship to life's realities. Braun, on finding himself met with tenderness in the transitional space created with his analyst when he recalled his mother's non-embrace allowed him to create a manageable and useable relationship to his psychic deadness and then his mortality.

Perhaps it is reasonable to think of Winnicott's transitional space as the obverse of Andre Green's described black emptiness of the emotionally "negative space" mother. Angela fled from her "black hole" as she called it, desperate until the very end for holding by others in order to avoid it. Braun could sit with his "greyness" as he called it, in the company of his "boatman" analyst, and transform his greyness into relatedness. To the extent that many people seem to think about death as something like their psychic death experiences, resolving those psychically dead places may greatly contribute to facing mortality.

Limitations

Many more questions await that cannot be addressed here. How does Freudian thought, most particularly about the death drive and conflict fit with existential maturity? Within the notion of existential maturity, how can we understand the internalization and decathexis that Freud described during mourning and its arrest in states of melancholia or complicated grief (Holland, 1998)? For instance, is the development of existential maturity hindered by, for instance, arrested mourning that serves defensively to keep the object alive (avoiding decathexis), perhaps because idealization or deidealization miscarried? And is there a cyclical process that includes the linear one (internalization, decathexis, moving on) that Freud described with a process of creating existential maturity that includes cathexis to internal objects in a way that mental representation of death allows?

Clinical Implications

In many regards, the psychoanalytic and dynamic care of people facing mortality is not different from other populations. Creating the holding environment, allowing regression to find the forward edge (Tolpin, 2002), using transitional space to create understanding and new directions, reknitting the disjunctions left by trauma, all in the context of analytic tenderness, are the same. Further, psychoanalytic and dynamic care is aware in its very fabric of the importance of sitting with grief and sadness for being able to process and move on.

Yet many psychoanalysts are not exposed to clinical considerations of care for the dying or family of the dying. Awareness of what a dying person and their loved ones need – encapsulated in this chapter under the term existential maturity – can help therapeutic listening and holding as the patient does the work they need to. Many people can grow and develop to the point that they can fully feel their mortality-related difficulties without destabilizing, and their connections can be vital without being destructive. This chapter tries to outline the unique kind of meaning-making, traumatic rupture repairs, relationships, and oscillations that are entailed in developing existential maturity.

The analytic relationship when a person is facing their or another's mortality is distinctive. More work is needed to identify its elements. For instance, the work of dying almost always entails permission giving and blessing among loved ones – a feature that is little covered in this chapter and needs more consideration elsewhere. Other aspects of the unique object relations and transference/counter-transference features are noted in this chapter, such as the role of the analyst in accompanying the patient to death (Brenda Solomon, October 2020, verbal communication). As in all populations, the patient who has not experienced the needed type of relating before will find or create it if they have first experienced it in the therapeutic relationship. For Braun, for instance, revisiting the playground scene was enough like meeting at the acropolis (Brenner, 2012) for it to be mutative for his existential maturity and ability to work at that level with his family and friends.

Care for those facing mortality can also inform other dynamic care. One question that comes up in every treatment is: when is the patient ready to end? The case of Braun suggests that analysts may want to consider if the analysand has sufficient existential maturity. Perhaps existential maturity can be understood as the capacity that crowns an analysis, which may emerge or mature in the terminating phase, and is the culminating change that allows both parties to consider their work complete. Indeed, in Braun's case, perhaps termination and achieving existential maturity became a united journey.

Likely, the amount of existential maturity that can be fostered is related to prior object relationships, though they clearly do not need to be fully healthy for good work to be done near the end of life. Quite possibly, having been well analyzed before, as Braun was, can be of great benefit. However, others achieve important work too. The therapist will do well to have a sense for what can be expected from treatment, whether it is the less fulsome but still valuable work that Angela completed or the more fulsome work that Braun completed.

We therapists are routinely analyzed as part of our own training and we are adjured to stay in a consultation relationship because of the reality that without having done and continuously doing our own work, we cannot help patients to do theirs. In the same way, therapists are not likely to be able to foster a patient in matters of existential maturity without having worked on their own. Therapists should work on their own existential maturity – at least to the point that their own limitations do not interfere with helping their patient reach it. Further, psychoanalytic and dynamic work with people in this situation is intense - intensely rewarding and also draining. Therapists should go into this work mindfully; as with other forms of analytic work continued support from a peer or consultation group is important.

References

Ahluwalia, S., Reddy, N.K., Johnson, R., Emanuel, L. & Knight, S. (2020). Dyadic model of adaptation to life-limiting illness. *Journal Pall Med* 23(9).

Atwood, G.E. & Stolorow R.D. (1984). *Structures of subjectivity: Explorations in psychoanalytic phenomenology.* New York: Routledge.

Becker, E. (1973). *The denial of death.* New York: Simon & Schuster.

Bion, W.R. (1961). Attack on linking (ataques al "vincular"), ps. 308–315. *Rev. Psicoanál* 18(1): 70.

Bion, W.R. (1962). The psycho-analytic study of thinking. *Int Journal Psychoanal* 43: 306–310.

Bowlby, J. (1958). The nature of the child's tie to his mother. *Int Journal Psychoanal* 39: 350–373.

Breitbart, W.*et al.* (2015). Meaning centered group psychotherapy: An effective intervention for improving psychological well-being in patients with advance cancer. *Journal Clin Oncol* 33: 749–754.

Brenner, I. (2012). A new view from the acropolis: Dissociative identity disorder. *Psychoanalytic Quarterly.*

Brenner, K.O. *et al.* (Submitted). Toward a psychologically informed palliative care: Lessons learned from an interdisciplinary seminar of experts. *Journal Pall Med.*

Chochinov, H.M. (2011). *Dignity therapy: Final words for final days.* New York: Oxford University Press.

Clark, D. (2018). *Cicely Saunders: A life and legacy.* Oxford: Oxford University Press.

De Masi, F. (2004). *Making death thinkable: A psychoanalytic contribution to the problem of the transience of life.* London: Free Association Books.

Emanuel, L. (2020). Learning from chickens. *ROOM*, October.

Emanuel, L. *et al.* (2020). Therapeutic holding. Retrieved from www.liebertpub.com/doi/abs/10.1089/jpm.2019.0543.

Emanuel, L., Reddy, N., Hauser, J., Sonnenfeld, S.B. (2017). "And yet it was a blessing": The case for existential maturity. *Journal Palliat Med* 20: 318–327.

Emanuel, L., Handzo, G., Grant, G., Massey, K., Zollfrank, A., Wilke, D., Powell, R., Smith, W. & Pargament, K. (2015). Workings of the human spirit in palliative

care situations: A consensus model from the Chaplaincy Research Consortium. *BMC Palliative Care* 14(1): 29.
Erikson, E.H. (1982). *The life cycle completed*. London: Rikan Enterprises.
Freud, S. (1915). *Thoughts for the times on war and death*. The Standard Edition of the Complete Psychological Works of Sigmund Freud, Volume XIV. Richmond: Hogarth Press.
Freud, S. (1917). *Mourning and melancholia*. The Standard Edition of the Complete Psychological Works of Sigmund Freud, Volume XIV. Richmond: Hogarth Press.
Galatzer-Levy, R.M. & Cohler, B. (1993). *The essential other: A developmental psychology of the self*. New York: Basic Books.
Green, A. (1993). Die tote mutter. *Psyche – Z Psychoanal* 47(3): 205–240.
Holland, J.C., Breitbart, W.S. & Jacobsen, P.B. (Eds.). (1998). *Psycho-oncology*. Oxford: Oxford University Press.
Jackson V.A. et al. (2013). The cultivation of prognostic awareness through the provision of early palliative care in the ambulatory setting: A communication guide. *Journal Palliat Med* 16: 894–900.
Johnson, R., Hauser, J. & Emanuel, L. (2020). Towards a clinical model for patient spiritual journeys in supportive and palliative care: Testing a concept of human spirituality and associated recursive states. *Palliative & Supportive Care* 19(1).
Klein, M. (1935). A contribution to the psychogenesis of manic-depressive states. *Int Journal Psycho-Anal* 16: 145–174.
Knight, S.J. & Emanuel, L. (2007). Processes of adjustment to end-of-life losses: a reintegration model. *Journal Palliat Med* 10(5): 1190–1198.
Mackay, M.M. & Bluck, S. (2010). Meaning-making in memories: A comparison of memories of death-related and low point life experiences. *Death Studies* 34(8): 715–737.
Pargament, K. (2007). *Spiritually integrated psychotherapy*. New York: Guilford Press.
Petriglieri, G. & Petriglieri, J.L. (2020). The return of the oppressed: A systems psychodynamic approach to organizational studies. *Academy of Management Annals* 14(1): 411–449.
Robert, M. (2012). Balint groups: A tool for personal and professional resilience. *Can Fam Physician* 58: 245.
Shedler, J. (2010). The efficacy of psychodynamic psychotherapy. *Journal Am Psychol* 65(2): 98–109.
Solomon, S., Greenberg, J. & Pyszczynski, T. (2015). *The worm at the core: On the role of death in life*. New York: Random House.
Tolpin, M. (2002). Doing psychoanalysis of normal development: Forward edge transferences. *Progress in Self Psychology* 18: 167–190.
Winnicott, D.W. (1965). The maturational processes and the facilitating environment: Studies in the theory of emotional development. *Int Psychoanal Lib* 64: 1–276.
Winnicott, D.W. (1974). Fear of breakdown. *Int Journal Psychoanal* 1: 103–107.

# Chapter 9

How a Lack of Human Connection May Lead to Dehumanization and Addiction

José Alberto Zusman and Edward J. Khantzian

Dependence

Understanding the role of dependence in human development is no easy task. Initially, because when regarded from afar by an observer untrained in psychoanalysis, dependence, mainly in adults, is frequently and mistakenly associated with pathology. From the cultural point of view, a healthy human being is seen as a member of a species that transitions from dependence (infantile phase) to independence (adult phase). Even within the field of psychoanalysis, dependence is often understood either from the prevalent cultural perspective of a pathological presentation or, in the best of cases, as a risky regressive mode process useful mainly for treatment purposes. Freud in his article on "Further Technical Recommendations" already warned young analysts about the dangerous regressive position a patient occupied during his psychoanalytic treatment. In his words: "One best protects the patient from injuries brought about through carrying out one of his impulses by making him promise not to take any important decision affecting his life during his treatment" (Freud, 1914, p. 153).

According to Philip Flores, "dependency is not only a confusing and pejorative term, but reflects a strong bias in our culture that not only reflects our obsession with … independence at all costs, but also is not in line with the biological realities of our species" (Flores, 2012, p. 89). Flores's statement alerts us to the fact that an obsession for independence may subject us to more hardships than successes. To put it simply, we are not, nor will we ever be, independent. Basically, human beings need other human beings in order to develop their full human potential. According to Parens and Saul: "When we speak of dependence we mean the need each human has, whether child, adolescent, or adult, for a libidinal object relation in order to insure his optimal psychic functioning" (Parens and Saul, 2014, p. 9). In fact, we are dependent from the very beginning to the very end of our lives, or as Richard Gill puts it: "from the cradle to the grave" (Gill, 2014, p. xiii). Bowlby understands that

> dependency always carries with it an adverse valuation ... it has often happened that, whenever attachment behavior is manifested during later years, it has not only been regarded as regrettable but has even been dubbed regressive. I believe that to be an appalling misjudgment.
>
> (Bowlby, 1988, p. 12)

Perhaps because of that negative interpretation of dependence, Hermann, following the attachment theory, preferred to lay emphasis on the physical aspect of human connection when he used the term "clinging" to define a human "instinct" and "the urge to separate as a reaction formation against it" (in Greyskens, 2003, pp. 1520–1523). Likewise I here suggest that the concept of dependence (which is more comprehensive) should be seen as an "instinct" inherent to the human species and, as it will be better put below, independence as a reaction formation against it. Fairbairn might have been the first psychoanalyst to consider the fundamental aspect of dependence in human development. According to him, we exist on a spectrum of dependence, "the total dependence of the newborn takes a gradual path to the mature dependence of the adult personality" (Fairbairn, 2008, p. xii). Like Fairbairn, other well-known authors such as Kohut and Winnicott have also taken notice of the misconception surrounding the concept of dependence. In the words of Jan Tonnesvang:

> In *The Restoration of the Self* (Kohut, 1977) the understanding of maturity and autonomy as independency was replaced by an understanding of autonomy as mature dependency. Ever since, Kohut has understood human connectedness as ontological and dependency as a part of humanity instead of a sign of immaturity.
>
> (Tonnesvang, 2002, p. 154)

In the other words, autonomy, unlike independence, should be seen as a state of maturity in which we are able to make our own choices towards constructing a healthy life. Therefore we, as psychoanalysts, should try to help our patients reach a state of autonomy and not a fictitious state of independence. According to Winnicott: "Individual maturity implies a movement towards independence, but there is no such a thing as independence. It would be unhealthy for an individual to be so withdrawn as to feel independent and invulnerable" (Winnicott, 1986, p. 21). Or rather, still according to Winnicott, independence, if it indeed existed, would seem closer to pathology than to health. Independence should be seen more as a sort of reaction-formation aiming to hide our true unconscious dependent instinct demands. In this sense independence is seen closely related with the phenomena of dehumanization that may often lead us to addiction as will be shown below. To understand this aspect deeply, it is fundamental to have a notion of how the external and internal worlds may interact in the formation of our human identities and raise some doubts about the difficulties psychoanalysis has had in understanding this apparently simple complementarity.

The Internal and External Components in the Formation of Our Human Identity

Undervalued in the world of psychoanalysis, the external human and nonhuman environments are fundamental to the formation of our internal identities. A materially welcoming environment, together with healthy human connections may be of great help in shaping our human nature. In other words, from the very start, the infant must find a safe and welcoming environment, human and nonhuman, for her own wellbeing. This goes from the loving eyes of the infant's mother, to the soft and cozy blankets placed around her body to keep her warm and safe. Through his concept of holding, Winnicott highlights the importance of both emotional and real physical contact between mother and child. Here the concept of internal and external are joined together as developmental elements that can work as allies. He adds with his concept of transitional objects just how much we live, at least with more evidence during the initial period of our lives, in a hybrid landscape in which external and internal, human and nonhuman mix and complement each other. In Winnicott's words: "The infant can employ a transitional object when the internal object is alive and real and good enough. But this internal object depends for its qualities on the existence and aliveness and behavior of the external object" (Winnicott, 2005, p. 13). He then follows by highlighting the importance of time and bonding maintenance to this transitional experience. According to him:

> when the mother or some other person on whom the infant depends is absent ... [her] internal representation of her ... remains alive for a certain length of time. After that ... the memory or the internal representation fades ... the transitional phenomena become gradually meaningless [and] ... we may watch the object becoming decathected.
> (Winnicott, 2005, p. 20)

The loss of love connection with the external world or with its internal representations is a terrible menace to the formation of our self. Green, following the same line of thought, coined the concept of the "Dead Mother" where a live caretaker becomes decathected by the infant for his lack of affective presence and attunement (Green, 1997, pp. 208–209). That is to say that the child of a dead living mother will be a dead living child, a dehumanized being who can easily be seduced by connections with an inanimate object. Although Freud did not dedicate much of his interest to the mixing nature in our development, he has made allusion to this aspect with his concept of "Complemental Series" (1916/17) and went even deeper in his paper on "Mourning and Melancholia" (1917). One of the reasons for which this complementarity has proven difficult to be sustained in the psychoanalytic world may be due to Freud's frequent change of position in regard to this specific complementarity. For Freud the real world is sometimes seen as an ally to human development, and soon after presented as hostile and threatening to human existence. According to Loewald: "I believe that in Freud's thinking these two concepts of reality have never come to terms with each other, and without doubt the ... reality seen as hostile (paternal) power, has remained the predominant one for him" (Loewald, 1951, p. 12). In the psychoanalytic setting, the necessary convergence between external and internal elements has been emphasized by many authors, including Madeleine and Willy Beranger, for whom the physical spatial structure of the analytical setting is fundamental to the formation of a consistent connection in the relationship between patient and analyst. In their words:

> What we notice most immediately about the analytic field is its spatial structure ... An analyst does not develop in the same way if his armchair is placed a meter away from the couch or if the couch is placed in the middle of the room instead of being next to the wall. Moreover, the choice of a certain position by the analyst already reveals a particular internal attitude toward the patient.
> (Beranger and Beranger, 2008, p. 796)

The environmental aspect refers to the regular scheduling of the sessions, the physical installations of the consulting space, the furniture that the analyst and patient occupy, and even the lighting inside the office, depending on the time of the session. Many perceptive modifications felt as external may even be due to internal changes that occur at each session in light of the transferential/countertransferential scenario established between analyst and patient. A patient who, for example, arrives to his session more hostile than usual may project his hostility onto the analyst and consequently see him differently, more distant, showing disdain and contempt towards the patient. This may be a strategy either to protect the analyst from the patient's destructive rage or to protect the patient from the fury that is projectively seen in the analyst. The relationship between patient and analyst, via transference/countertransference communication is a dynamic, unconscious experience where two unique stories converge and connect, either repeating an old scene or creating a new story yet to be defined. Patients who arrive significantly traumatized by their past history may arrive to treatment trying to recreate with the analyst the sources of their internal pain as a way of communicating them without having to resort to words, either because they have not yet made the translation or because it may turn their experience into something even more painful.

Clinical Case I

Helen is a beautiful woman of around 30 years of age who was referred to me by her clinician after she attempted suicide by cutting her wrists. She was single and had a very poor social life. Though she dated frequently with a variety of different men, she sustained no emotional connections with them. When she arrived in my office, I was surprised by her coldness and by the obvious effort she put into maintaining her elegant appearance. She seemed to be eager to impress me by describing her professional success, which was really quite remarkable. My impression was that she came ready for a confrontation wearing an invisible yet noticeable armature. She was so keen to make herself appear powerful that I asked her what she was afraid of. She smiled sadly and responded:

> I'm afraid of everything and nothing. To begin with I didn't want to be here. I came just because I would be hospitalized by my father if I didn't. I don't want to go through that again. I've been hospitalized once before and it didn't do me any good. I hated it.

When I asked her if I could be helpful in any way she began telling me her life story. Helen recounted that she was the only child of an exceedingly vain mother and very aggressive and distant father. She said:

> In fact I don't think anyone ever really cared about me. My parents' idea of keeping me company was to take me to gatherings with their friends in fancy restaurants around the city. They dressed me up all pretty but they never spoke to me. I felt like they were showing me off in a window display. It was tedious. I don't remember them ever playing with me. They gave me toys and chocolate and everything necessary so that I would keep to myself in silence without bothering them too much.

As she said nothing about her suicide attempt, I decided to ask her directly about it. Helen replied that she didn't care much for this story. It didn't mean much for her. She said: "If you want to know what I think I will tell you, no big deal, too much fuss for nothing." Her apparent indifference gave me the impression that she wanted to show in actions what she was trying to tell me in words. And so she said: "I don't need you or your help. I really don't. I never had help when I needed it. I'm a survivor. I know how to live on my own. I never tried to kill myself. This is bullshit."

Somewhat bored, she carried on talking about how everyone was wrong about her. When she tried to cut herself, she did it because she wanted to ease her internal pain, not to die. She wanted to feel the pain because the pain made her feel alive. Physical pain didn't hurt. The pain was her friend. She also said nonchalantly that on several occasions she had almost died from cocaine overdoses and alcohol poisoning, but that she also did those things to feel alive without having to be with people or to rely on them. She said that what she really could not stand was the tedium and emptiness of her life and that is why she had to be in movement all the time, which was good for work purposes. She then said, in a sarcastic way, that she also had a "food dealer," a man who worked in a market close to her home where she used to go whenever she was sad or lonely. There she would binge on food, eating whatever she could find until she could not even breathe properly. In her words: "At these times it is as if I had a hole inside of me that cannot be filled. It's awful. I don't feel full. I feel ill and when I do I know it's time to go home." The next day she would have a "moral hangover," feeling like her binge had negatively affected her appearance, about which she cared so deeply, especially since she considered her attractiveness one of the few positive points about her.

My impression was that because she was incapable of forming stable and trusting bonds with other people, she turned to several types of addictive behaviors with drugs and non-drugs. Although very different in their genesis and evolution, they shared many commonalities. According to Wurmser: "they all are used to provide external relief for an internal urge of overpowering driveness" (Wurmser, 1974, p. 825). That external relief creates the impression to the addict that they live in a world apart where they were invulnerable or unreachable, protected against disappointments or sorrows inherent to the human condition. That attitude was obviously detrimental to her development and drove her even further away from building the human connections she so desperately needed.

Having this in mind, I told her I wanted to see her five times per week. She laughed with disdain and responded:

> You really need my money, don't you? OK, it makes no difference to me, I am rich, but if it matters to you I will come, but if I cut myself this time it will be your fault. I have nothing to lose. Good for me, bad for you.

Helen's treatment suffered a number of setbacks. She was quite suspicious and sensitive to any changes in my breathing, the sound of my voice, my wardrobe or when I would take time to travel (when I was, after all, spending her money), my occasional tardiness, the separation over the weekends (showing how much I truly did not care for her). Helen, for her part, was never late, nor did she ever miss a session. She liked to tell me that no matter what I did, I would never be able to get it right. It seemed like she was always trying to create an environment of competition in which her victories against me were used to tear me down and to prove how people were simply not reliable. In fact, on several occasions I felt I had lost confidence in my abilities to treat her. The feeling was terribly unpleasant. On one particularly difficult day for me I commented on the feeling of discomfort I sometimes felt when we were together. Surprisingly she smiled and responded, with a certain air of triumph:

> That's life, doc. You've got it. This is the way I feel all the time. It's funny that you mention that today because I haven't been well for a long time and I thought you never noticed. You always had that analyst's way of talking, cold and distant. I never felt we were close. I was even thinking about cutting myself again. Who knows if I did something like that we could feel something together for once?

My understanding was that she was searching for a peculiar connection with me, one in which she felt the physical pain while I suffered the emotional trauma of the story; one pain complementing the other.

When I asked her why she hadn't said anything to me about it up to that moment. She said: "You see me every day and don't notice? Am I obliged to tell you what is happening with me? Are you blind or can't you see me?" As the session drew to a close, she fell silent. I waited a while and then remarked that her last comment made it seem like she thought I was acting just like her fancy, cold parents. She responded: "Just like everybody I have ever met in this damn world." She remained silent the rest of her session. So did I.

For almost the whole first year of treatment Helen complained and blamed me for everything that made her suffer in her daily life. It was terribly unpleasant for me but I understood that I had to hold on to her so that she could be sure I would be there for her if or when she ever needed me. For me, that appeared like the sound of the many emotional scars she carried from several disappointments she suffered earlier with very significant figures of her life. Gradually she began to show some fruitful changes. She stopped cutting herself; she began to relate to food in a more appropriate way but continued to sporadically use cocaine and alcohol. In the middle of the second year she began to tell me when she was planning to binge on food or alcohol, to use drugs or when she had recently used them. I had the impression that we were beginning to share some intimacies between us. This gave us a chance to begin relating her behavior of retreating from human contact to her feelings and thoughts. Gradually she began to come to her sessions in a more casual way and started talking more loosely. One day she came in, lied down on the couch and spoke with some tiredness and some hope:

> Listen, I don't want to fight anyone anymore. I need help. I can't carry on living in the war I have lived in always thinking people are going to hurt me. Either I change or I'd rather die. I have no other option.

Helen cried in a heartfelt and moving way. Although the feeling was one of sadness, I felt a sense of relief at her outburst. I was touched and commented that it seemed she had shed some of her armor, and that she was running the risk of exposing herself to me and asking for my help. I told her I thought that was a positive sign we were developing a good personal connection and that I appreciated her confidence in me. She replied: "Maybe, but I still don't feel comfortable in this position." When I told her that it is sometimes necessary to feel a certain level of discomfort in order to be able to change, she smiled and said:

> Up to now you have always been wrong, but today you got it right just a little. You know this gives me some hope, but let's not do like AA says. Let's try not to take it one day at a time. I need much more than that.

Three years later, Helen, who had not attempted suicide or binged on food or used drugs during that time, showed up to her Monday sessions and seemed to be in good spirits. I mentioned this to her and she responded:

> This weekend was a good one. I met a new guy. He seems like a nice person. He is from abroad. He is different. I felt he was really seeing me. I don't know. He made me feel visible. I felt good. Today I woke up a little cheerful.

When I told her that maybe between us a true connection had also existed, for some time, she began to cry and said: "You know, everything is all very confusing. I'm happy. At least I think I am, because I never have been. But I'm scared to death. If I need to can I call you?" I answered that of course she could, and that she had always known that. Helen smiled. So I said: "You might be afraid that I'll use the fact that you feel better so that I don't have to worry so much about you and can give you less attention. The old story of turning the good into the bad." She said she wasn't so sure of that anymore because she now trusted me. She remained silent. I did not interfere. I knew that at that moment she was not feeling abandoned. It seemed to me she was turned inwards, thoughtful, perhaps carrying on a conversation with me within herself. She appeared to me to be better, and I felt more comfortable in session with her. An image came to mind of a small child abandoned on the beach who was no longer scared, not because she had found her way, but because she had trusted in a human adult who had taken her by the hand so that they might walk together, a person she could finally depend on.

A year later she got married and went to live abroad. In her last session she seemed pleased and so was I.

Addiction

Addiction is the end product of a heterogeneous condition marked by severe deficits in early object relations and/or overwhelming conflicts due to the internalization of these early bad experiences. For Leon Wurmser: "there is no sharp line between specific addictions and addictive behavior in general except for the contingencies of the physical aspects induced by specific drugs" (in Volkan, 1994, p. xvi). That is consistent with Joyce McDougall, for whom the addictive object may be anything invested as "good" in spite of its dire consequences (McDougall, 1985, p. 66). The addictive object could be any object or activity chosen that is taken or injected (e.g. drugs) or done (e.g. behaviorally) in exaggeration that puts life at risk despite the knowledge the person supposedly has about it. Brian Johnson understands this defense act as: "a psychological system, referred to as denial (which) is created around harmful behavior" (Johnson, 1999, p. 797). For Johnson: "If there is no denial there is no addiction." In addition to that, Bower et al. say that: "as well as those behaviors that specifically involve the ingestion of substances, there are a number of other compulsive behaviors … that are also often said to have 'addictive elements' or 'addictive like' qualities" (Bower et al., 2013, p. 7). Addiction is a symptom and as such it is a compromise formation in the sense put by Charles Brenner (1982) that points to something that didn't properly work in the early emotional connection between the person and his human environment. Bower et al., summing up Johnson's paper from an object relation perspective state that this viewpoint was developed by Fairbairn, Klein and Winnicott and that it assumes that: "all humans are object seeking from birth and that these internal object relationships are … based on actual experiences of parents or caretakers as well as unconscious phantasies about them" (Bower et al., 2013, pp. 5, 6). I here suggest the existence of two lines of possible development in man, one following the triad of dependence, human connection and humanization that goes in an opposite direction from another formed by independence, dehumanization and addiction. The first triad leads to health, the second to pathology. As written above, dependence is a human instinct and independence is a reactive formation and therefore the one line of development that follows our true nature will naturally lead us to a healthy pattern of living and the other, being a mistake from the beginning, will bring the person closer to pathological states. This closely follows Winnicott's concept of true and false self (Winnicott, 1965). Krystal (1974, 1975, 1997), Khantzian (1999) and Khantzian and Albanese (2008) given the intense necessity an infant feels towards her caretakers, mainly during the initial stages of childhood, stress that failures in the relationships between caregivers and the infant may cause severe damage to the personality formation of the person. We are so dependent on the connections we establish in the real relational world that we unconsciously create an internal representation of that world that enables us to survive and be our true selves in life. These internal mental representations of the external human and nonhuman world are constantly reinforced by new connections. For Joseph Sandler and Bernard Rosenblatt this representational world functions like a stage upon which the scenes and dramas of inner life are enacted and influence all of our future paths (Sandler and Rosenblatt, 1962, p. 134). Throughout this complex process some representations endowed with high affective importance become stable objects fundamental for the acquisition of trust in our self and in our object relations (ibid., p. 132). This is similar to the concept of object constancy, which, according to Kevin Volkan, "refers to the mental representation of a loved object which remains internally within the mind of the infant ... whether or not it needs to be satisfied" (Volkan, 1994, p. 68). Object constancy is a representation of a good object. Margaret S. Mahler, Fred Pine and Anni Bergman understand that this stable internal representation would have to include not only good objects, but also bad ones being therefore more consistent and cohesive. In their words, it "implies the unifying of the 'good' and 'bad' object into one whole representation" (Mahler et al., 1975, p. 110). Fairbairn, on the other hand, following another perspective, understands that we only internalize the negative objects and relationships in the external world and that our relationship with real and gratifying objects need not be internalized. For Fairbairn, internalization would function as a protective shield against bad relationships so that the good ones could be preserved as idealized experiences. Whatever the case, an addict never reaches this point of internal stable organization. Unable to attain harmony with another human and lacking an environment of sufficient comfort, a person from the early stages of development will search for a survival strategy. That is to say, in Green's words, that the child of a dead living mother will be a dead living child, a dehumanized being who can easily be seduced by connections with an inanimate object. Dehumanization may come with the feeling of invulnerability and detachment seen only in patients who have been internally or externally traumatized and are badly damaged. In adulthood this may also happen when faced with an internal or external traumatic experience through the reactivation of their transitional objects (Vamik Volkan in Volkan, 1994, p. 73). Addictive objects function in this way, and in doing so help the addict to find shelter against dysphoria (Khantzian, 1999; Khantzian and Albanese, 2008) and internal pain due to lack of self and affect regulation (Krystal, 1974, 1975, 1997). However, unlike true transitional objects, objects of addiction do not lead human beings towards the path of healthy development, nor do they create spaces of creativity. Unable to stand the pain life may bring, the addict finds himself in an impoverished, desolate and concrete internal scenario, resulting from the severe damage to the process of abstraction and symbolization (Wurmser, 1974, p. 837). According to Shure: "As in the case of splitting and omnipotence, dehumanization is basically a primitive defense. Its presence is frequently a signal that relatively regressed transference/countertransference tensions have become activated" (Shure, 1984, p. 39). There is an emptiness of the human affects that causes the person to stop caring for her (self) or for others (objects).

At the end of the day, dehumanization is a situation in which the representations of people and the healthy connections made with them may be substituted by a false connection with inanimate things. As a species we are born human but unlike hominization, which is part of our inescapable biological development, *humanization* is an achievement that corresponds to a subjective process of development which may or may not be acquired through contact with other human beings, and that may be compromised by internal or external traumatic situations. In other words, severe external traumas such as experiencing hostile parenting or internal traumas such as the loss of an important loving bond may cause a person to arrest their human development. Addiction emerges as a desperate strategy to manage the dehumanized and impoverished conditions in which a person loses their self-esteem and compassion, caring little for others or themselves. In Fairbairn's point of view, drugs will have at first a seductive presentation and second will reveal their frustrating aspect. The addict caught in this wheel mill of contradictory experiences may end up adopting a state of indifference (dehumanization) in which the only thing that matters is surviving each moment, non-sequentially, in a concrete, cold and tedious way. Perhaps that explains the maxim uttered by self-help groups such as AA, in which life should be taken "one day at a time," with no consideration for yesterday (no guilt) or tomorrow (no frustration).

Clinical Case II

Sally is the youngest of four sisters. She came for treatment eight years ago, at 45 years of age, because of her feelings of depression that were intensified by the recent death of her father. She had a very contentious marriage and although having tried very hard, they were unable to have children. Her own mother had not wanted her when she became pregnant, and attempted to secure an abortion on many occasions. However, she was finally forced to stop searching because her pregnancy had advanced too far. As soon as she was born, her mother became severely depressed and Sally had to be sent to her grandmother's house for about three months. She was not breast-fed. Her mother, probably due to her fragility, dedicated herself only to her own needs and cared little about the rest of the family. Her father had to work hard all day long and when at home had to care for her mother who was always depressed and needed a great deal of attention. In our first session she hardly spoke. But just on the second she arrived in a furious state, saying that I had been very aggressive to her, that she realized that I had almost physically assaulted her and that she had felt very scared. She continued saying that she didn't know why I had disliked her so much and that she would only continue her treatment with me because she had no option. My feeling was one of perplexity. I had not felt at all the way she described but quite the opposite. I had felt sorry for her and for her pain. On the other hand, at that point her distorted perception by her transference was so powerful I felt like she wasn't seeing me at all and there was nothing to do to convince her she was welcome in our sessions. Later, as she began to tell me her story, I had the impression that in our initial sessions she was enacting the beginning of her life when she had been so rejected by her mother. In my mind I had a picture of a baby that after waiting far too long for food and affective shelter entered a kind of "protesting mode" in which she could no longer accept what she so desperately needed because she had to complain so furiously for being left alone. It took a long time until she stopped being so aggressive and could listen to me. Once she came and said:

> I don't expect anything from anyone because I always get disappointed at the end. I learned that my fate was to be lonely from the beginning. I don't have and never had a proper family. We were a bunch of people together each one fighting to survive. No one ever talked with anyone. My father was weak but at least he was a good man. Now I have nothing. I have a husband but the scene is almost the same.

She told me that she spent her entire day in her room because the world was awful and at least in there she felt safe. She didn't go out much because if she confirmed how bad the world really was she would not be able to stand it. In her room she would eat all day long, alternating between taking the sleeping pills and stimulants she was able to buy from a nearby pharmacy without a medical prescription. She would also watch all the soap operas she could. For almost two years I mostly listened to her, since she gave me no room to talk. Although we agreed to have five sessions a weak, she missed most of them. When she eventually came to a session she wouldn't let me say very much and complained repeatedly about her past sufferings and loneliness. All those times I felt like I was set aside and left as an observer in the process. I tried to tell her that but she wouldn't listen. During this period, our sessions were mainly focused on her rage and the methods she adopted to protect what she felt was good in the world by staying away from it. On one occasion she came to me and we had the following conversation:

SALLY: I want to know what you see in me. I have always wanted to know if people saw bad things in me that kept them distant. There must be something very wrong with me, otherwise what would explain my own mother rejecting me even before I was born.
THERAPIST: When you first arrived here you also thought I rejected you and I didn't.
SALLY: But you did, but I don't want to talk about this again because this makes my angry and you don't admit it.
THERAPIST: Perhaps what you see as evil in you is your rage for having been rejected. You don't consider that you also might have rejected people around you in response to not trusting them.

SALLY: That may be, but why should I. On the other hand I try to be nice, I only say these awful things to you. I am always nice to others. I keep giving presents to people around me. But it simply doesn't work.

My impression was that Sally was slowly trying to develop a means to create a new story for herself. In our third year of treatment her relationship with me had become more stable and she rarely missed a session. She continued having a lot to say, but she no longer silenced me; she listened to the things I had to tell her. In her sixth year of treatment, she managed to stop taking pills, she lost weight and as her relationship with her husband improved considerably, they decided to adopt a child. By that time she came in with a new fear:

SALLY: You know this might seem crazy but I am scared to death that my kid will like my husband more than me and that I will be excluded. They might just not need me anymore.
THERAPIST: Was that the fear you had when you first got here - that I wouldn't like you because my preference would go to all of my other interesting patients who could satisfy me more?
SALLY: I think you are right. I am always afraid that there won't be a place for me. On the other hand, I don't want to be in my room, with my food and my pills anymore. I don't have to be in a womb where I had to be supplied with the toxic food full of rage and rejection my mother gave me.
THERAPIST: Perhaps now you might feel confident enough, strong enough to reach out to the world and build your own first family in which you feel welcome. Perhaps you might find yourself in a position that you may even have enough in you to feed your son with food, love and everything he may need.

How Can the Analyst Help?

For Bower et al., "Given the high incidence of addictions, its perhaps surprising that the psychoanalytic literature on addictions is sparse, with a few notable exceptions" (Bower et al., 2013, p. 1). Perhaps this can be explained by the enormous difficulties an analyst has to face when dealing with patients that are so difficult to treat and that may cause so much disturbance in the analyst and in the analytical field. In order to treat patients who are suffering from addiction, the analyst must flee from traditional analytical distance. According to Khantzian: "therapeutic modes of impassivity and strictly interpretative approaches are not in the order of the day and indeed can be counterproductive" (Khantzian, 2015, p. 10). Their first and most important task for the analyst is to create a stable, trustworthy connection based on a human bond. Through this the patient may acquire the opportunity to encounter or reencounter a living human being within themselves; an experience that can help them remember or develop their own humanity. This is not an easy process. Nor is it a rapid or painless one. In both clinical cases described above I tried to make clear the discomfort felt by the analyst when put in a position of an "excluded observer," which has been well described by John Steiner (2011, p. 86) where the analyst has to tolerate what he calls "the observing transference" in which the analyst is only allowed to "comment and observe" without being part of the main affective scene. On the other hand, it was made apparent the discomfort the patient feels when their relationship with the analyst grows stronger and they begin to show some intimacy. Initially, the analyst must face a specific countertransference by which the subject of the analyst is regarded with suspicion and distance. The analyst may even feel "the pressure to be drawn into making extra-transference interpretations, commenting on the patient's relationships" (ibid., p. 87) outside the clinical setting. An addict may rely more on inanimate objects than on humans. Humans fail them while inanimate objects do not, the latter being at their disposition and under their control. That is why at first the analyst must be able to withstand the emotional reactions to being treated as an inanimate thing. An addict does not seek happiness; they cling to some kind of connective element that makes them feel alive, even if that involves self-mutilation or injecting toxic substances into their veins. Despite the analyst's understanding these actions as an attack on the creation of an analytical connection, it is necessary for them to keep in mind that the patient undergoing treatment, when faced with his own pain, has no other option but to react in this manner. According to Khantzian, an addict keeps their dysphoria under control by using drugs. It may also be relevant to consider that the relationship with the analyst could ameliorate the discomfort of their unpleasant feelings of dysphoria (Khantzian, 1999). Treating addicts successfully requires that analyst and patient bear the bitter taste of abandonment, boredom and emptiness, together. Given their disdain for life, addicts care nothing for others, which only increases the constant threat they feel that the connections they make with the analyst will fail. In the words of Luis Rodrigues de la Sierra, the addict: "not only deals in a very complex way with his feelings, but is also capable of provoking disconcerting and confusing feelings in the analyst" (in Bower et al., 2013, p. 82). The unconscious communication via transference–counter-transference is very relevant, especially when dealing with addicts. In truth, for the addict, this human connection may often be seen only as the sophistication of their pain in the face of yet another potential frustration. According to Fairbairn, drug use reedits this trajectory, from the seduction of a release from the pain to a greater sense of frustration once the effects of the drug have worn off. I would add that the same could be said about behaviorally addictive elements such as gambling or food binging. It is a long road until the analyst is rendered as a human object of constant representation. Nevertheless, even the slightest disappointment can have grave consequences to maintaining this connection, and menace the structure of life itself.

Some Final Remarks

This chapter suggests the existence of two lines of human development that do not have a fixed organization, and can therefore be altered usually with the help of a deep bonding circumstance such as the one that may be lived in the analytical field. As described above, a healthy development is represented by the triad "dependence, human connection, humanization" and an opposite devitalized and degraded version of this line is formed by the triad "independence, dehumanization, addiction." Although all addicts may be different in their clinical presentations, they may have in common a severe lack of human connection in the beginning of their lives. The entrance of drugs on scene considerably changes clinical aspects, treatments and outcomes, but behavioral addiction (e.g. food addiction, sex addiction, gambling, etc.) may also present their clinical particularities and may offer serious threats to life. Dependence, although often overlooked, is a universal human trait and as such is central to the development of a healthy life. On the other hand, independence, which is usually held as a human goal, is a reactive formation that if pursued with too much obstinacy may lead to feelings of failure, frustration and may ultimately lead to the realm of dehumanization and addiction. Psychoanalysis may be of great help to people who desperately need to establish or reestablish a human connection in order to understand themselves as human beings. The connections made, though tenuous at first, may be enough to give voice to an addict's silent scream from their inner void. As trust develops, an addict's inner turmoil can finally be heard and understood by another human being with whom it is possible to establish a real human connection; one that gives meaning to the particularities of the human adventure to live and to enjoy being alive.

References

Beranger, M and Beranger, W. (2008). The Analytic Situation as a Dynamic Field. *The International Journal of Psycho-Analysis*, 89(4): 795–826.
Bower, M., Hale, R. and Wood, H. (Eds.) (2013). *Addictive States of Mind*. London: Karnac.
Bowlby, J. (1988). *A Secure Base*. London: Basic Books.
Brenner, C. (1982). *The Mind In Conflict*. Connecticut: International University Press.
Fairbairn, W.R.D. (2009). *Then and Now*. Edited by N.J. Skolnick and D.E. Scharff. New York: Routledge.
Flores, P.J. (2012). *Addiction as an Attachment Disorder*. New York: Jason Aronson.
Freud, S. (1914). Further Technical Recommendation. In *The Standard Edition of the Complete Psychological Works of Sigmund Freud*, Vol. 12, p. 153. London: Hogarth Press.

Gill, R. (2014). *Addictions From an Attachment Perspective*. London: Karnac.
Green, A. (1997). *The Dead Mother. On Private Madness*. London: Karnac.
Greyskens, T. (2003). Imre Hermann's Freudian Theory of Attachment. *International Journal of Psychoanalysis*, 84(6): 11529–15517.
Johnson, B. (1999) Three Perspectives on Addiction. *Journal of the American Psychoanalytic Association*, 47: 791–815.
Khantzian, E.J (1999). *Treating Addiction as a Human Process*. New York: Jason Aronson.
Khantzian, E.J. (2015). *A Psychodynamic Understanding of Addiction: An Overview*. Paper presented at 49th IPA Congress, Boston, MA.
Khantzian, E.J. and Albanese, M.J. (2008). *Understanding Addiction as Self Medication*. Lanham, MD: Rowman and Littlefield.
Krystal, H. (1974). The Genetic Development of Affects and Affect Regression. *Annual of Psychoanalysis*, 2, 98–126.
Krystal, H. (1975). Affect Tolerance. *The Annual of Psychoanalysis*, 3: 179–219.
Krystal, H. (1997). Self Representation and the Capacity for Self Care. In D.L. Yalisove (Ed.), *Essential Papers on Addiction*. New York: New York University Press.
Loewald, H. W. (1951). Ego and Reality. *International Journal of Psychoanalysis*, 32: 10–18.
McDougall, J. (1985). *Theaters of the Mind: Illusion and Truth on the Psychoanalytic Stage*. New York: Basic Books.
Mahler, M. S., Pine, F. and Bergman, A. (1975). *The Psychological Birth of the Human Infant*. New York: Basic Books.
Parens, H. and Saul, L.J. (2014). *Dependence in Man*. London: Karnac.
Sandler, J. and Rosenblatt, B. (1962). The Concept of the Representational World. *The Psychoanalytic Study of the Child*, 17: 128–145.
Shure, R. (1984). *Counter-transference Enactment*. New York: Jason Aronson.
Steiner, J. (2011). *Emerging from a Psychic Retreat*. New York: Routledge.
Tonnesvang, J. (2002). Selfobject and Selfsubject. *Progress in Self Psychology*, 18: 149–166.
Volkan, K. (1994). *Dancing Among the Maenads*. New York: Peter Lang Publishing.
Winnicott, D. W. (1965). *The Maturational Processes and the Facilitating Environment*. London: Karnac.
Winnicott, D. W. (1986). *Home is Where We Start From*. New York: W. W. Norton & Company.
Winnicott, D. W. (2005). *Playing and Reality*. New York: Routledge.
Wurmser, L. (1974). Psychoanalytic Considerations of the Etiology of Compulsive Drug Use. *Journal of the American Association*, 22: 820–884.

Chapter 10

Psychoanalytic Approaches to the Skin Patient

Jorge Ulnik

Somatic diseases and symptoms are explained in medicine in terms of a change in the interplay of organic tissues and blood cells, cytokines, neuropeptides, etc. in a previously homeostatic stage. The loss of homeostasis is thought as being caused by external stimuli like infections, physical stimuli like trauma or radiations, or at best neurogenic inflammation produced by stress affecting the "real" body. The first sensation in mind is that the "real" body is like a machine and the medicine is the science and the technique for its repair and maintenance.

Working with hysterical patients, Freud discovered that the hysterical conversion is an affection of the representation of the body, not of the body itself. This affection is related with the sexual life that resides in an erotic body, that does not coincide with the anatomical body and that has predestined erogenous zones, being the skin the most important of all of them.

During my hospital career, the medical-psychological interconsultations were the ones that attracted me the most, because they allowed me to discover the history that is hidden in the patient's body. Generally, a story of suffering, conflicts, emotions and pain.

We are unconsciously motivated by two mistakes: one is the belief that the suffering is in the body and always comes from it. Thus, what we see, what we prove, what we touch, explains all pain. The second mistake is the belief that the body suffering without material substratum is only a phantasy. In other words: a suffering with a material pathology would be completely explained by it. And a suffering without a material pathology would be different and less important and real than the first one.

What I was proving over and over again was that this dichotomy was false. The skin is the limit between the inside and the outside, the screen for the projection of emotions, the organ of communication and the surface for the reception of stimuli. By means of it, the fissure that separated the perception from representation, the psyche and the soma, the internal and the external world, was blurred. The specialists who asked for consultations most frequently were dermatologists, and in practice with skin patients I was greatly helped by reading Freud, who gave it the status of "erotogenic zone par excellence." Referring to the skin in the

DOI: 10.4324/9781003167679-11

Freudian work does not exclusively mean to speak of the skin as an organ and its eroticism, but also to speak about the functions and diseases of the skin; the drives that are originated in it; the action of touching and its consequences, as well as contact in general and its relationship with contagion; the relationship between the skin and the gaze, the skin and the identity and, lastly, about the Ego and the functions of boundary, surface, protection and perception as well.

The experience of working with skin patients introduced me also to the world of tattoos and self-injury.

As if it was a two-way street, I was able to better understand the skin patients after approaching the comprehension of tattooed and self-injured people, but the opposite way also occurred: I observed mixed cases in which a true allergic reaction, after being successfully treated with steroids was substituted by a self-injurious behavior, which generated very similar lesions in the same locations as the allergy. As if both phenomena – eczema and self-inflicted lesions – carried out the same message.

Witnessing patients with vitiligo lesions tattooing themselves on top off the lesions to cover the "holes" left by the disease, I could understand that the tattoos and self-injuries can function as substitute marks or patches that fill in other kinds of holes and voids: emotional, existential, or identity voids. That led me to a more benign conception of tattoos than I had. Tattoos are damage to the skin, but they can fulfill a necessary function for some people, and they can even be a solution – albeit a prosthetic one – for certain lacks of origin marks. Thus, the case of a boy who was begotten by means of a fertilization technique consisting of the donation of ovules that were later fertilized with his father's sperm. He hurt himself without remedy, until he got a tattoo shared with his mother. He could not have the genes in common, but they had the tattoo, and with that he stopped cutting his skin, a behavior that unconsciously fulfilled the function of making identity marks that he lacked.

By understanding why an allergy arises after a traumatic event, a psoriasis after a separation, a vitiligo after a dramatic scenic change, etc., psychoanalysis advances in many fields. It advances in the understanding of body language of the early childhood, of the symbiotic bonds of some attachment disorders, of the massive identifications, of the role of the own image and that of the others in the formation of the human psychism. It learns to listen to the "dialogue" between the skin and the gaze and explores, beyond the skin, the mind–body relationship at stake in our patients suffering. This relationship has always interested thinkers and clinicians from the most diverse branches of knowledge throughout the world.

What is a Skin Patient?

First of all, we are all skin patients. No one is exempt from suffering from an allergy, pimples, acne, a skin rash from a medication, a sunburn (later on an actinic keratosis) or some chronic inherited disease.

It is also true that traumatic life events can be triggers for a variety of skin diseases, including those with autoimmune, inflammatory, viral, etc. characteristics. On one occasion, I had to assist a young boy with a very severe atopic dermatitis. The disease began at age 5, after an accident in which his parents and a brother died. It was almost impossible not to think that his disease, with its genetic condition and allergic characteristics, was unrelated to the trauma of the accident and the subsequent orphanage situation. What is more, he had outbreaks every time his caregivers traveled abroad

Once the disease appears, the skin patient will be the one who feels "marked" by his or her disease. And that mark will often be associated with a feeling of dirt, humiliation, stigma (in ancient times the stigma was the penalty of aesthetic mutilation). All this without control.

An essential characteristic of the skin is that it is an organ that can be seen. Therefore, the skin patient will look and feel looked at. And this will bring into play a pulsional exercise and a dialogue between the skin and the gaze. This pulsional exercise will be able to follow several destinies, some of which were called by Freud "pre-repressive": the turn against the own subject and the transformation in the opposite. And so, voyeurism and exhibitionism, sadism and masochism, love and hate will alternate in the relationship of the subject with his skin.

There will also be a series of affections that will be at stake in the skin patient: one of them is shame, and the other is envy. It is enough to have a skin disease to become aware of the beauty that the skin possesses … the skin of the other.

Along with these affections there will be a feeling of discomfort. Like the one you feel when you put on an itchy outfit, which is too small or too big, which you don't like, which bothers you in some way.

And you will also feel anger: against fate, against others, against yourself or against your own skin, which you will want to tear off, clean, polish, erase, paint in a thousand ways. We had said that the skin is an organ that can be seen. Well, the skin is also an organ that can be touched. And that characteristic, both passive and active (because I'm the one who touches and I'm the one who's touched at the same time), will make it the inflamed, bloodshed, flaked scenario of that rage and that struggle.

The Encounter between Psychic and Somatic

In "Pathways of mutual influence," Freud suggests that every modification in the field of biological needs and functions can have an influence upon the erogeneicity linked to the particular organ that carries out these functions. And, likewise, every alteration in an organ's erogeneicity can also affect its biological functions (Freud, 1905a). In this way, highly erotized skin, or in contrast, scarcely stimulated skin, could become ill in different ways: generating itching, becoming infected with herpes, showing blisters or even eczema and other inflammatory reactions. What is more, as Spitz has noted (Spitz, 1965), sometimes the contradictory maternal stimuli to a child can participate in the eruption of an eczema.

Life jumps from one side to the other time and time again over the abyss between psyche and soma. Accompanying such jumps from the therapy space is risky, but possible. It is as if when facing a hole in the fabric, instead of regretting because the edges cannot be joined, we sort of mend it. To do this, we need access to a transindividual, transdisciplinary and savage way of thinking and processing.

Transindividual because there are many patients with clustered families, symbiotic relationships and symptoms that seem related to the stories, beliefs and customs of the ancestors. Thus, there is a transgenerational transmission. Transdisciplinary because it is necessary to work as a team and be willing to have the other specialist's point of view modify and enrich your own, generating a more complex, creative and new (or novel) approach. And when we say savage we do not refer to an inferior or aboriginal thought, but as Lévi-Strauss says (Keck, 2005), we refer to a type of primitive thought in its pure state, as we once had in our evolution and that then we were able to overcome. This type of thinking puts in the foreground the restoration of the meaning of the disease and its place in the history and dynamics of the patient and his family. Furthermore, it relates – erasing partly its borders – the body, the internal world, the external world and the other with whom we relate.

Meanings don't always manifest themselves in the same way. Sometimes the quantitative factor is essential, and the level of stress or the strength of emotions don't allow the significant to play its role. Thus, inspired by Charles Peirce's semiotics (Deladalle, 1996), we are allowed to state three different forms of somatization:

- The index somatizations are the ones that occur as a consequence of stimuli that are above a threshold. For example, a reaction to a high and unspecific stress. They are consequence of a quantitative excess. They are *indicating* the excess.
- The iconic somatizations are the ones that *imitate* the stimuli. Maybe mirror neurons could have an essential role in this kind of somatic response.
- The symbolic somatizations are the ones that *symbolize* an idea, a feeling or a complex scene. They imply a high range process, complex imitation, and an unconscious but stronger intention of the subject to communicate.

There could be different ways in which the body reacts to indicate, to imitate or to symbolize our inner world of emotions, thoughts and representations.

Levels of symbolization

From my point of view, the eternal debate about the meaning of somatic disorders and the symbolic capacity of psychosomatic patients, when posed in dichotomous terms (they symbolize vs. they don't symbolize) obliterates the knowledge of the existence of different levels of symbolization. It does not matter if the most basic level does not deserve to be called symbolization, or if our conception in layers or levels does not prevent a sharp distinction between the symbol and the sign. What matters is that analogies and equivalences take on an enormous weight when the distance between representation and perception shrinks.

There is a painter whose art works show us the coexistence of symbols and signs: Giuseppe Arcimboldo. His paintings evoke different levels of objects. For example:

Level 1 A pear. (When looking very closely at the nose of a portrait.)
Level 2 A nose in the face of a man. (When we go further and see a face.)
Level 3 Someone's known face: Haubsburg Emperor Rudolf II. (When comparing the gestalt of fruits with a portrait of the emperor.)
Level 4 The summertime. (When realizing that all painted fruits and vegetables grow in the same season.)
Level 5 Vertumnus (When we reach a higher level of abstraction.) In Roman mythology, Vertumnus is the god of seasons, change and plant growth, as well as gardens and fruit trees. He could change his form at will, using this power.

The combination of insignificant elements produces the birth of the meaning. But the combination doesn't wear down the creation of the meaning: if you draw away your perception you can engender a new meaning. You can combine the elements at another level.

If we extrapolate this to our job as psychoanalysts, that's where we can make good use of Arcimboldo's technique. For example, when we purposely combine the body, the world and the other – the three dimensions that Green considers fundamental of representation (Green, 2010) – we "make" a meaning where perhaps before there was none. To do this we use as elements the "fruits," and the "objects" of the patient, including his natural parts, both healthy and diseased. The fact that the product of that combination, made of displacements and analogies is a meaning that does not come as a whole from the patient's psyche, does not mean that it is alien to him or that it does not function as a therapeutic tool.

Thus, there is a staggering of articulations not only taking part of our complex psyche but of our complex biology. Combining different levels of symbolization, patient and doctor establish equivalences: sometimes, the equivalence of *being*: "the lymphocyte *is* a killer" and sometimes the equivalence of *making*. S. Connor has mentioned a woman with an eczema lesion in the same place where her mother had the tattoo of a concentration camp (Connor, 2004). The image of the concentration camp tattoo on the mother's hand and the story of suffering that has been told to her daughter, *makes* the daughter's suffering equivalence which, as a result, also makes the eczema lesion in the same place. In this context, "makes" means "composes" the same as music is composed or created.

An Experience of Interdisciplinary Approach to Patients with Psoriasis

People usually go to a therapist's office for psychotherapy sessions. But the referred skin patient goes to the psychotherapist with the same goal as he or she goes to the doctor: to get rid of the skin disorder. So when the psychotherapist suggests that psychotherapy sessions are needed and the outcome is not guaranteed, the patient is disappointed.

Patients often express objections such as anticipating that psychological and psychoanalytic treatments will generally be long; that they are not told in advance when therapy will end; that the frequency of sessions is too high (even if they are once a week); that health insurance plans do not cover psychoanalytic treatments; that the cost of psychological interviews and sessions should be added to the overall cost of treatment, etc. (Ulnik, 2016).

How to deal with all these difficulties?

Freud said:

> When I set myself the task of bringing to light what human beings kept hidden within them, not by the compelling power of hypnosis, but by observing what they say and what they show, I thought the task was a harder one than it really is. He that has eyes to see and ears to hear may convince himself that no mortal can keep a secret. If his lips are silent, he chatters with his finger-tips; betrayal oozes out of him at every pore. And thus the task of making conscious the most hidden recesses of the mind is one which it is quite possible to accomplish.
>
> (Freud, 1905b)

A psychosomatic approach and the words mentioned above encouraged me to put into practice the experience of joint treatment (dermatological and psychoanalytical) of patients with psoriasis. The patients who come to our clinic have severe psoriasis and are treated in a state of art dermatology combined with a psychoanalytic approach. Upon entry, the patient consults with a team of a dermatologist and a psychoanalyst. During this consultation the patient "shows" his troubles to the dermatologist or "speaks" about them or about related life events to a psychoanalyst.

What the Psychoanalyst Hears When the Dermatologist Sees (Ulnik, 2008)

It is surprising how patients talk while being physically examined, or when they relate their experience with prescribed medications. In addition, there are patients who begin their consultation by talking about their family, work and general emotional problems, while others are quick to "show" and describe what they exhibit. During the joint attention, the first ones are approached by the psychoanalyst first, and then by the dermatologist. The latter, on the other hand, are questioned about their life or triggers after being physically examined.

Listening to the patient's speech when he talks to the dermatologist, the analyst should consider different levels of symbolization. Patients have a singular relationship with their body and with their disease. The common phenomenon of "personalization" of lesions while describing them allows the analyst to hear what is in patient's inner world, under the skin, and projected on it. Sometimes, when a mourning process is at stake, the analyst can perceive the "shadow of the object" (Freud, 1917) that is over the skin. Listening complaints, he/she can perceive the "suffering envelope" (Anzieu, 1987).

What the psychoanalyst hears in the doctor's consulting room allows him to infer that there are unconscious factors which have a part in:

- The motive and the time of consultation.
- The self-destructive patterns of behavior that make the disease worse.
- The kind of complaint or suffering that will be privileged by the patient.
- The acceptance or rejection of a treatment or of a medicine.
- The location of the lesions.

What the Dermatologist Sees and Hears (Ulnik, 2008)

When the psychoanalyst asks and the patient speaks, the dermatologist also hears and in certain cases this can modify his therapeutic criterion.

Psoriasis is a disease that improves with a highly varied number of treatments and it is up to the dermatologist to decide which. If the cure obtained with medical treatment is not definitive, the dermatologist faces different options, and the wider the variety of medications and the less he knows about his patient, the more difficult the decision becomes.

On the other hand, both the favorable and the adverse effects will have a "symbolic efficacy" (Lévi-Strauss, 1958) that the psychoanalytic interview could determine. For example, the odor of a product is not described as an adverse effect; however, it could be if the patient to whom it has been prescribed feels dirty and contemptible in advance, or if he is an obsessional neurotic who is concerned with cleanliness.

Likewise, it has also been seen that some patients only obtain the caresses they want from their wives by making them put the creams on for them.

It is not the function of the dermatologist to offer any interpretations. However, during the psychoanalytic interview new channels of expression are opened.

His usual experience is that he has to obtain quick and visible results so as to ensure that the patient comes back to see him. But with the work in common with the psychoanalyst, links beyond what is visible are developed and they ascertain continuity and allow the dermatologist to opt for schemes that, despite the fact that they do not promise immediate or spectacular effects, are far safer and more feasible, and are very effective when the cure is understood as *a process* and not merely as a result.

The unconscious factors, as well as the personality traits, can have an influence not only on the better acceptance of a particular medication, but also on a better therapeutic response.

Caresses can increase cream's curative power, and not only make it more tolerable.

It is not the same to tell a patient that his lesions will be erased, that they will disappear or that they will be cleaned. Words maintain some of their ancient power even today and "physicians practise psychotherapy without the intention of doing it, or even without being aware of it" (Freud, 1904).

It was seen that those patients with a higher degree of masochism subjected themselves to, and even seemed to need, highly aggressive treatments.

Many patients come to see us saying that they know we will not cure them, and yet still they come. We believe that this attitude corresponds to a repetitive compulsion: what is repeated with the doctor is the hope of receiving the love promised in childhood followed by the subsequent disappointment of abandonment, indifference or cruelty.

The experience of interdisciplinary work with psychoanalysts and dermatologists working together was very well accepted by the patients. Some joined groups and others followed individual treatment. Patients with alopecia areata, vitiligo, atopic dermatitis and self-inflicted lesions also showed interest in the interdisciplinary psychosomatic approach.

The Meaning in the "Real" Body: Allergy, Identity and Skin

The psychoanalyst Joyce McDougall mentions herself as a case (McDougall, 1989). When she was a child, she developed urticaria each time she visited her grandmother in New Zealand. Although her family thought that it was an allergy to the milk of the Jersey's cows, she suddenly was aware that she had allergy every time she faced her family environment, dominated by her grandmother, who had been imposing her will to everybody. When she could be separated from the grandmother's influence, the urticaria disappeared. This example suggests that a person could be "allergic" to another person, even if the allergens of the other's skin are not present.

Allergy is a very fertile field of psychosomatic research. Marcelo, a 40-year-old patient with atopic dermatitis, had the characteristics that were named by Gieler the "allergics to everything" (Harth et al., 2009): He was raised in a depressing and demanding family atmosphere. After a time of analysis, he talked about a grandfather who was the exception: playful, happy, tender, and dedicated to him. He was strongly attached to his grandfather, who died suddenly. Since then he has not approached emotionally anyone else. Then, he lost his dog, and this event marked the permanent closure of his emotional world. If alexithymia didn't start at that time, at least we can say that after that it worsened a lot and remained fixed. At the beginning of the treatment, he expressed himself through the skin. His friends called him "the redskin" as a nickname stressing in that way his identity problem. Through his therapy process, I saw that his perception of the environment was distorted. The peak moment happened when he received an invitation from his boss who gave him a ticket to see the final of soccer Championship cup, in which his favorite football team was one of the competitors. His team won the match and obtained the cup. All fans were exultant! Nevertheless, as the final was played on a rainy day, he was worried about the rain, the wet sensation, the rubbing with other people – the stadium was full – and he wanted to go out before the Olympic round, to avoid all the excess of skin perceptions.

His comments – "How wet I was!," "A lot of people around touching me!," "I could hardly breathe!" – revealed how a disease modifies and conditions the environment perception. Thus, the therapy only works if we help the patient not only to express his feelings with words, to re-build his Ego image and his significant bonds but also a to get a new environment conception.

To change the environment conception we have to consider what D. Anzieu called "formal representations," apart from word-representations and thing-representations (Anzieu, 1987).

The formal representations are the representations of line, of plane, of surface, of sphere, of the position of the body in space, of envelope, of container, internal-external, etc.

For the baby there is no difference between space and the objects that inhabit it. In consequence, when one moves an object, one moves at the same time the part of the space in which the object is. And the child himself is an object that occupies part of space and that can be pierced by another part (Anzieu, 1987).

Alteration of formal representations would lead to confusions between the notions of inside-outside, and one's own and alien, which would be a permanent source of conflict and anxiety. The theory of formal representations could also explain the alteration in the concept of distance shown by patients and their disruptive behavior of abrupt detachment or abandonment of relationships that were starting to become close due to an affective approach.

It is as if the approach were experienced as an imminent danger of fusion. This reflects a problem in the construction of one's identity and body boundaries. Allergy would seem to be the somatic manifestation of this same problem. The disease manifests itself as an exaggerated defense reaction against antigens that when recognized, and being somehow "familiar," are treated as strangers. The intense itching and consequent scratching would seem to be attempts to pull out that familiar/ stranger that has come into contact with the self. When atopic dermatitis becomes chronic it becomes a mark of identity, but a "sensitive identity" based on pain, touch, look or any other input coming from the sense organs.

In one session Marcelo came full of rage and feeling itchy, telling me that a short video was sent to his workmates. In it, his face appeared edited to the body of a character in a cartoon in which he was dancing with others. Each character had the face of one manager of the enterprise. He found out who was the author of the video and called him. Very angrily, he told him: "If I see my face in another video and it is yours, I will immediately fire you!"

I showed him that his phrase was ambiguous: "the video with my face is yours" means: "you are the author of the video with my face," but at the same time "my face is yours" Means "my face is your face," "you have owned my face," "my identity is yours,"[1] "You have taken my face/identity and have done something with it."

As he was suffering a deep narcissistic wound, I told him something to re-build his Ego: "You didn't take into account that they joked only with the most important and powerful guys of the enterprise. Please, tell me, who are the others?" He learned he was not his workmate, he was not the only one in the video, they (the other managers) weren't him and he was an important manager. Everyone has his own face. As a result of the intervention, he decided to take the video out of his mobile and save it in another mobile that he used only for work, and the itch stopped.

After a long time of treatment, he is being called Marcelo by his workmates, he expresses his emotions verbally, and it's been two years without outbreaks or unbearable itching. Recently, in a party where there were old and new friends of his, a girl asked him: "By the way, I don't understand why your friends call you 'redskin'?"

We can continue mentioning cases with close connections between diseases and life histories, but ... what about evidence?

Paraphrasing Steven Connor:

> It is generally easy to agree with specialists in psychosomatics that the whole body is a sensitive marker of different mental and physical states. What is less easy to accept, or even perhaps to understand, is the claim that the body allows the more or less direct picturing of those mental states, as images or allegories.
>
> (Connor, 2004)

The Three Dimensions of Representation and the Mimetic Moment

According to A. Green, the field of representation extends over three different spaces: the body, the world and the other.

To transform the representations that we are building we have to invest them. If we refuse to give them value, or if they are too painful, we fail to suppress them or free ourselves from their domination, repression fails and the difference between representation and perception is abolished (Green, 2010). When this happens, the world, the body and the other are intermingled, activating original semiotic sources. "The meaning of objects is experienced as inseparable from the sensual qualities that can be perceived on its surface." "Therefore, the place of objects and the constitution of outer space as a reflection of the interior create a spatial equivalence without discrimination" (Green, 2010).

While tattoos are made by means of the will and on the contrary, diseases are not a product of the will, they both have in common what we might call the "mimetic moment." In it, perception and consciousness coincide. It occurs when trying to capture, materialize, and be the narrative starting point of a feeling, a situation lived, a person with whom the subject relates, an object of reality, etc.

The mimetic moment is usually duplicative of a visual impression that being unfinished seeks to be completed; it's like the print of a threat; a mark of a sexual identity; a reversal of the inside and the outside, the permanence of a childlike self that persists eternally, etc. It can give meaning to an experience without a name.

The Mirror Neurons and the Skin

The mirror neurons discoveries help us to give a biological support to our theoretical work about the mimetic moment or about the imminent danger of fusion that some patients have when they feel closeness with someone else (Iacoboni, 2009).

Mirror neurons are brain cells that help us to understand the actions of other people simulating in the brain the same actions through the activation of motor plans. Reproducing face's motor movements during emotions, mirror neurons help us to feel what other persons feel, through some neuronal connections with the insula and the limbic system. These cells appear to create a sort of intimacy between the Ego and the other helping us to feel the same as others (Iacoboni, 2009).

Mirror neurons discoveries support conclusions about the close bond between perception and action. For example, they activate themselves when a person: kicks a ball, sees someone else kicking a ball, sees a ball prone to be kicked or hears the word "to kick." So, perception is very important even when it is only word perception. And by means of mirror neurons, what a person perceives prints his body via mirror neurons – Insula – Limbic system (Iacoboni, 2009).

But ... What will be printed? Where? With what ink? Could the skin be the paper?

Iacoboni (2009) says that in an experiment with MRI, when showing facial expressions of babies to a mother, they trigger a cascade of automatic brain answers of simulation that recreate real interactions between mother and baby.

What kind of cascades of brain answers, but also hormonal, and why not, inflammatory reactions triggers on our "Connor's patient example" – mentioned above – the tattoo of her mother?

The body, the external world and the other with which we have a bonding are three well-defined entities with very precise boundaries of separation. However, from the discovery of the mirror neurons, Ramachandran suggested that:

> [W]hen someone is touched you can empathize with the other person, activating your mirror neurons as if you were touched on the same place of your body. *But you do not actually experience the touch. There is a feedback signal from touch and pain receptor on your skin, preventing you from consciously experiencing the touch. But if you remove the arm you dissolve the barrier between you and the other human being and when he or she is touched you literally experience the touch. The only thing that is separating you from him is the skin. Remove the skin, and you dissolve the barrier between you and the other human being (...) If a person with a phantom leg sees another person who is touched, he feels his phantom leg to be touched. But the astonishing thing is that if he feels pain in his phantom leg, he sees another person who is being caressed and he feels pain relief in his phantom leg ...*
>
> (Ramachandran, 2009)

Following Ramachandran's statements, we can imagine that a patient could develop a lesion in the same place where her mother has a concentration camp tattoo, because probably she is feeling pain or refusal feelings located in or towards the same place where her mother's body is tattooed. How many times would her mother have thought: "I wish I could eliminate this tattoo"? Or: "It is important to conserve and show it as a message for the future of human rights"?

Thus, the tattoo could be a familiar and foreign image at the same time. As allergy is a reaction of rejection to something, which is in certain way familiar and strange, the eczema in the daughter's wrist makes sense. What should be a simulation of mirror neurons turns out to be a reaction of the skin's immune system.

"The Ego and the other are melted in an inextricable way through mirror neurons" (Ulnik, 2016).

The Identity and the Other; the Death on the Skin

Peter has an appointment with the dermatologist after his session. While he undresses for the physical exam he leaves a pile of scales on the floor. The dermatologist asks him how he is doing and Peter, pointing to the scales on the floor, replies, "look, there I am."

What Peter sees in his own scales is himself, as if he were another who leaves traces everywhere. This other "presence" is disavowed by his dermatologist and his psychoanalyst, who just hoover the floor, as Peter's wife always does, and put Peter's "other me," which, incidentally, is torn to pieces, in the rubbish bin. I learned this from a patient with psoriasis who spoke of her divorced mother saying *"If I moved in with Dad, Mum would fall to bits,"* while her skin came off in small pieces. As if it were a molt, the shedding of the skin allows the materialization of the ominous phenomenon of the double.

Steven Connor in his *book of skin* gives us some clues about the meaning of the shedding scales skin: mentioning the Michael Jackson's "Thriller" video he says that "in our mortuary imagination, the dead are not absent or decomposed. They are ragged, held together by shreds and patches." As a compromise between skin and fur or skin and hair, rags have a libidinal charge. Hair is immensely important as a way of focusing and amplifying skin sensation. As well as tangled hair, ragged clothes and shedding scales skin seem to signify "a body alert or awoken to touch," soliciting touch. But at the same time "an unnatural life resides in the raggedness" of the walking dead and the shedding-scales skin. Both are "the busy life of decomposition, a dying that walks." As in a snake, the skin is also the sign or our transformability, our ability to become other, as well as our identity, our ability to persist and survive in becoming other. Furnishing disguise or transformation, skin becomes a means of preservation (Connor, 2004).

Symbiosis and Mind–Body Dissociation: Technical Considerations

Mr. Areyouthere had been evolving his psoriasis for 18 years without any remission. He belonged to a clustered and incestuous family in which cousins married each other. When after a few years of psychoanalytic treatment he improved from his illness, two significant events occurred. On the one hand, his wife, who seemed to be the healthy one of the couple, became ill of the skin, evidencing that there was a "body for two" between them (we could say *psycosomatique a deux* paraphrasing *folie a deux*). And on the other hand, when he saw himself without injuries, he seemed to miss the disease. At night, repeating a childish behavior he had with his mother, touching her in the bed where they slept together, he stretched his arm to his legs looking for psoriasis lesions and between dreams said: are you there? Are you still there?

With her skin reaction, the wife of Areyouthere made it clear that symbiotic couples are always constituted by a complicity of both members of the symbiosis, and that although one of the two is the one who suffers from the disease, the other remains healthy because he has deposited it in the first.

The body–mind dissociation is a form of immobilization and control of the symbiosis that implies the coexistence of a mind with a logical – rational organization with a body that experiences the affections intensely without identifying them as such.

These people generate in others fear, uncertainty, anger, reactions corresponding to affections, etc., which they cannot take charge of because they cannot integrate them into their psychism:

> The mind of these patients has a strong logical-rational organization and affections are directly lived in the body. They have to learn to discriminate and represent them (perceive them) in the area of the mind, and for this it is necessary to overcome the dissociation of body–mind.
> (McDougall, 1989)

For this reason, one possible technique is to point out to the patient his or her affections by showing him or her physical behavior, and then give a name to that emotion. This is a double-edged sword that requires an interpretative art: assisting dermatological patients I have understood that it hurts them to feel transparent and misinterpreted, as for example when looking at them with alarm because they have an outbreak, others tell them: "What happened to you!?" whereas they didn't want to tell anything. Usually, the others attribute feelings to them or assume they are unwell without first listening to them. Besides, it is common that patients have a part of the self that feels and another that reveals itself against that, because the self that feels cannot avoid giving to see what it feels, even when the other part of its self would not want to show it, at least consciously. Therefore, the way of interpreting the bodily messages to convert them into emotions must be playful, indirect, analogical, similar to the way we sometimes interact with small children when we attribute life and feelings to their dolls. For this it is useful to work projectively: talking about what happens to a third party, who may even be a pet, we can nominate the feelings that the patient is feeling without realizing it or accepting it completely.

Miss M, 28 years old, suffers from severe erythrodermic psoriasis and lives with her parents and younger sisters. She has suffered from her disease since early childhood and is completely dependent on her family. For some time now, she has been expressing her desire to go and live on her own. She describes everything she is going to do, how happy she is, makes plans, buys objects for her future home, but while she says this she starts to get worse from her skin to unbearable limits. The analyst listens to a person who, in his mind, is very happy to go live alone, but at the same time he sees a person who, with her body, says, "Don't let me go live alone, because I'll break into pieces, I'll dust myself! The father and the rest of the family ask the analyst in anguish: do you really believe that M is in condition to go and live alone?" She got all the Doctors and psychologists in the institution thinking: – *"How on earth are you going to go and live alone in this state, if you are to be admitted to intensive care!"*

Alluding to a similar situation of a patient named Katia, Green states: "the less internal space she has to use, the more she is forced to use the external space, but this space is not neutral, it is obvious that it is loaded" (Green, 2010).

Another aspect to consider is the current state of maturation of the patient's Ego. If we place in front of his mirror – which is us – an eroticized identity and the patient still does not know if he is a man or a woman, if he is a human being or an animal, or what he is, the idealized image of the mirror turns out to be an anticipatory image that precipitates an aggravation, because it is an image that is ahead of the patient's possibilities of being able to integrate and assimilate it.

What improves the patients is that the emotions and the thoughts come together, and that they go in synchrony and pace because what makes them sick is that they dissociate and run emotions and thoughts at different rhythm accentuating the psychosomatic dissociation.

The dissociation body-mind is not only that, but also a dissociation body + external world on one side and mind on the other, because the body is part of the external world, in which there is also the analyst and the analyst's body. That is why Green says that the dimensions at stake are the body, the world, and the other (Green, 2010). And Liberman argues that symbolization fails when these dimensions cannot be properly differentiated from each other (Liberman et al, 1982).

The difficulty of separation is impossible to overcome if the external world – which includes one's own body and that of others, including the analyst's – is an indiscriminate, clustered syncidia and is not integrated into the mind

For example, a patient of mine with psoriasis in his legs had difficulties in walking and standing up. Once he got rid of the psoriasis in his legs, his varicose veins worsened and he got an infection. His difficulty to stand up and walk remained unaltered. Did he only have psoriasis or a legs difficulty to continue moving forward with his legs along his life? I saw several psoriasis patients with metabolic syndrome who didn't go to the beach using their skin disease as an alibi. Once the skin was healed, the obesity replaced the psoriasis as the excuse to expose their body in front of others.

The Skin and the Gaze

The subject of the gaze is important both from the theoretical framework and from the clinical point of view (remember that the drive to see can be a subrogation of the drive to touch).

The caresses, the holding, the thermal stimuli, of pressure and pain, and the cares given in the cleaning, leave traces of importance in the psychic evolution of the individual. The punishments received and the dermatitis of childhood, also contribute to increase the particular erogeneity that the skin has "par excellence." But it should not be forgotten that the skin is different because it is visible and photosensitive. This characteristic determines a function of communication and affective expression that is very important in social relationships.

The body scheme[2] is built with the complex articulation of many elements among which tactile and proprioceptive sensibility, language allusions referring to one's own body and that of others, and the specular image in which we recognize ourselves, related in turn to the images imposed on us by culture (Schilder, 1958).

When this articulation is not properly produced, identity can try to be sustained by a single element, independently of the others (Ulnik, 2008). For example, a subject may feel that he exists only because of his image.

In "New paths of biology," Portmann (1963) says that animals do a great job in maintaining their appearance, and that contrary to popular opinion this work is not justified only by mimicry, protection from predators or the need to attract the sexual partner for mating. In "Mimicry and legendary psychasthenia" Roger Caillois (Callois and Shepley, 1984) argues the same. Apparently the external forms and drawings would be "made" for a certain eye, so that they would be directed phenomena.

Portmann calls "directed phenomena" those that are directed to a receiving structure and "own phenomena" those that try to self-represent the animal or the living form that produces them (Portmann, 1963).

Both in patients with identity disorders and in those with self-destructive masochistic tendencies, the idea that everyone should see their horrible injuries is in line with this characteristic of living beings to develop drawings on the skin either as phenomena directed at a receiver, or as self-representative phenomena of their own.

It could be argued that contrary to what is being suggested, patients do not show but on the contrary tend to hide their injuries, pretending that nobody sees them. But the very fact of hiding, often beyond what is necessary, is nothing more than evidence that in his fantasy the patient feels exposed "in front of everyone and for everyone" [*Erga omnes*] (Ulnik, 2008). This feeling explains the lack of differences in the effect on the quality of life – pointed out by Ludwig et al. (2009) – between skin patients with visible lesions and those with hidden lesions.

Regardless of the location of the lesion, the feeling of exposure and the prejudices to which the dermatological patient is subject are similar. Skin diseases, it seems, cause feelings of exposure and constraint regardless of the part of the body involved, because it is intimacy that is affected, and the skin disorder always threatens it, avoiding privacy. The intimacy transcends the location: a person may have genital psoriasis and another person may have it only in the elbows, but both may feel affected their intimacy in the contact relationship with the other. This is how F. Sampogna et al. (2007) note that the sexual difficulties of patients with psoriasis do not correlate with the genital location or the severity of the disease, and Magin and others (Magin et al, 2010) studied the speech of patients through semi-structured interviews and mentioned cases in which sexual concern is associated with fear of the other crosses the barriers and not exclusively with the aesthetic aspect or location. The latter was corroborated in a study carried out by us at the University of Buenos Aires (Ulnik, 2013).

Whatever their appearance, race or condition, in front of a fellow man we recognize him and we place ourselves with respect to him. We thus obtain reciprocal recognition. However, the field of reciprocity of the gaze is conducive to deception, both because of the concealing action of the mask – hence today's adolescents use the term "mask" to refer to those who live by and for appearances – and by the presence of the lure that attracts and confiscates the eye.

Much of the horror that skin disease produces is that it transforms the sufferer into a non-resembler. The blood, the fat, the flesh without the covering that is the skin do not work as a mirror where we can recognize ourselves. Hence the rejection of the skin patient that we so often observe in society.

The dermatologist faces this horror by moving the unrepresentable to a known terrain. To this end, he names and classifies the lesions according to their shape and location, most of the times with diagnostic and therapeutic sense, but in others he only aims at avoiding the anguish by attributing to the lesions the shape of a coin, a drop, a medal, etc., precisely where the stain emerges as an alteration of the normal. In fact, the dermatologist takes the patient as his object, he being the subject who looks at it. But while his eyes are captured by the lesion, he is at the same time the object of the patient's gaze. The lesion "looks at him" and the patient observes him (Ulnik and Ubogui, 1994, 2000; Ulnik, 1998). The disease acts as a decoy (Ascher, 1980).

In humans there also exists a function that we could call the veil or the appearance that consists of representing something on an imaginary plane tending to the concealment of the true being that escapes all representation.

Lacan mentions the example of Zeuxis and Parrhasios who were competing to see who could paint better. Zeuxis painted on a wall some grape clusters of such realism that, acting as a lure, some birds rushed over them. Parrhasios was the winner, however, because he was able to paint a veil on the same wall, so similar to a real one that Zeuxis said impatiently: "Come on, show me now what you've done back there" (Freud, 1895).

Lacan continues: Unlike the birds,

> when one wants to deceive a man, one presents him with the painting of a veil, that is to say, of something beyond which he asks to see […]. Only

> the subject – the human subject, the subject of desire that is the essence of man – is in no way totally imprisoned, unlike the animal, in this imaginary capture. In it he orients himself, how, insofar as he isolates the function of the screen, and uses it.
>
> (Lacan, 1964)

The screen fulfills a function of mediation, and at the same time, of *trompe-l'oeil*.

The less subjectifying the gaze of the parents has been, the more anxiety will manifest itself in the scopic field, and the predominance of the image can cause the failure of the mediating function of the screen.

As we said above, there is a kind of dialogue between the skin and the gaze. From this last one, a subject can feel loved and recognized, or on the contrary, he can come to doubt his own existence, and look for his identity by all possible means. In the "Project of Psychology for Neurologists" (Freud, 1895), Freud emphasized the importance of the peer complex in the subjective constitution, in recognition, empathy and reciprocity.

When a child is not recognized, when the gaze of his parents goes through him as if he were transparent, or when they look at him as though he were an inanimate doll, or when, upon his image, that of a dead relative is over-imprinted, the child becomes a curtain, as if behind or through him there existed the scene that the Other wishes to see. He then offers, like the painter, his function as a stain:

> Do you want to see beyond me? Well, look at this! And while you look at the nothing that I am, I will observe you.
>
> (Lacan, 1964)

Final Words

We are all exposed to an external environment that is both hostile and a provider of the love and contact we need. We also experience, at times, the sense of inner emptiness, the endless search for meaning in our lives, the bitterness and drive of unfulfilled desire.

Skin disease could become a means of emotional expression, a surrogate form of identity, a defense against the mental illness or psychological suffering a patient feels unable to face. The psychoanalytic perspective contributes to the dermatology practice providing diagnostic dimensions, unconscious dynamics, fruitful explanations and therapeutic strategies that help the physician to recognize structural psychological needs of their patients and the multiphacetic qualities of the skin: Screen to the outside of our emotions, our skin is like a mantle that represents and contains us, but that does not get to touch what is beyond what we can reach; means of contact with the others, it is the most exposed to that the rubbing leaves indelible marks to it, and those marks, as if they were words, carry our suffering written; erogenous zone par excellence, it is the one that shrinks not only with the passage of the years but also with love disappointments.

Notes

1 Two-year-old children generally talk in 3rd person while they are building their own Ego.image. Sami Ali has a theory about the face in which the baby first doesn't have a face, then has the face of his mother and finally has his own face, but it is felt as coming from the other (M Sami Ali, 2010).
2 Note that Schilder's concept of body scheme is used and not F. Doltó's concept of body image, because while the former includes the biological body, the latter excludes it (Doltó, 1990).

References

Anzieu, Didier (1987) *El Yo-piel*. Biblioteca Nueva.
Ascher, J. (1980) Être Peau-Cible. *Psychologie Médicale*, 12(2), 439–444.
Callois, Roger & Shepley, John (1984) *Mimicry and legendary Psychastenia*. MIT Press.
Connor, Steven (2004) *The book of skin*. Reaktion.
Deladalle, Gérard (1996) *Leer a Peirce hoy*. Editorial Gedisa.
Doltó, François (1990) *La imagen inconsciente del cuerpo*. Paidós.
Freud, Sigmund (1895) *Project for a scientific psychology*. The Standard Edition of the complete psychological Works of Sigmund Freud (ed., trans. James Strachey), vol. 1. Hogarth Press.
Freud, Sigmund (1904) *Psychotherapy*. The Standard Edition of the complete psychological Works of Sigmund Freud (ed., trans. James Strachey), vol. 7. Hogarth Press.
Freud, Sigmund (1905a) *Three essays on sexuality*. The Standard Edition of the complete psychological Works of Sigmund Freud (ed., trans. James Strachey), vol. 7. Hogarth Press.
Freud, Sigmund (1905b) *Fragment of an análisis of a case of hysteria*, The Standard Edition of the complete psychological Works of Sigmund Freud (ed., trans. James Strachey), vol. 7. Hogarth Press.
Freud, Sigmund (1917) *Mourning and melancholia*. The Standard Edition of the complete psychological Works of Sigmund Freud (ed., trans. James Strachey), vol. 14. Hogarth Press.
Green, Andre (2010) "Thoughts on the Paris School of Psychosomatics." In *Psychosomatics Today*. Karnac.
Harth, W., Gieler, U., Kusnir, D. & Tausk, F. (2009) *Clinical management in psychodermatology*. Springer.
Iacoboni, Marco (2009). *Las neuronas espejo*. Katz.
Keck, Fréderic (2005) *Lévi-Strauss y el pensamiento salvaje*. Ediciones Nueva Visión.
Lacan, Jacques, (1964) *The four fundamental concepts of psychoanalysis*. Karnac.
Lévi-Strauss, Claude (1958) La eficacia simbólica. In *Antropología estructural*. Eudeba.
Liberman, David, Grassano de Piccolo, E., Neborak de Dimant, S., Pistiner de Cortiñas, L. & Roitman de Woscoboinik, P. (1982) *Del cuerpo al símbolo*. Kargieman.

Ludwig, M. W. B., Oliveira, M. S. O., Müller, M. C. & Moraes, J. D. (2009) Qualidade de vida e localização da lesão em pacientes dermatológicos. *Anais Brasileiros de Dermatologia*, 84(2), 143–150.

Magin, P., Heading, G., Adams, J. & Pond, D. (2010) Sex and the skin: A qualitative study of patients with acne, psoriasis and atopic eczema. *Psychology, Health & Medicine*, 15(4), 454–462.

Mamhud, Sami Ali (2010) *Corps réel, corps imaginaire*. Dunod.

McDougall, Joyce (1989) *Teatros del cuerpo*. Julián Yébenes.

Portmann, Adolf (1963) *New paths in biology*. Harper & Row.

Ramachandran, V.S. (2009) The neurons that shaped civilization. Retrieved from www.youtube.com/watch?v=l80zgw07W4Y.

Sampogna, Francesca, Gisondi, P., Tabolli, S., Abeni, D. & IDI Multipurpose Psoriasis Research on Vital Experience Investigators. (2007) Impairment of sexual life in patients with psoriasis. *Dermatology*, 214(2), 144–150.

Schilder, Paul (1958) *Imágen y apariencia del cuerpo humano*. Paidós, Biblioteca de Psiquiatría, psicopatología y psicosomática.

Spitz, René (1965) *The first year of life. A psychoanalytic study of normal and deviant development of object relations*. International Universities Press.

Ulnik, Jorge (1998) *Psychological factors affecting psoriasis*. 5th European Congress on Psoriasis and 7th International Psoriasis Symposium, Milan.

Ulnik, Jorge (2008) *Skin in psychoanalysis*. Karnac Books.

Ulnik, Jorge (2016) Psychoanalysis in psychodermatological diseases. In Klas Nordlind & Anna Zalewska-Janowska (Eds.), *Skin and the Psyche*, 187–222. Bentham Science Publishers.

Ulnik, Jorge (2013) Factores subjetivos en la sexualidad, el contacto y la calidad de vida de pacientes con psoriasis. *Anu. Investig. – Fac. Psicol., Univ. B. Aires*, 20(2): 301–307.

Ulnik, Jorge & Ubogui Javier (1994) La escucha del psicoanalista y la mirada del dermatólogo. *Actualidad Psicológica*, 19(207): 16–19.

Ulnik, Jorge & Ubogui, Javier (2000) Psoriasis as affective expression means. *Dermatology + Psychosomatics: Abstracts of 8th. International Congress on Dermatology and Psychiatry*, 1: 39–40.

Chapter 11

The Balint Group

The Arc of the Enduring Bridge between Psychoanalysis and Medicine

Randall H. Paulsen and Don R. Lipsitt

> The importance of Michael Balint's work lies in the application of psychoanalytic knowledge by the general practitioner to the treatment of emotionally disturbed patients who never consult a psychiatrist.
>
> (Knoepfel, 1972, p. 379)

In the 1970s, the documented incidence of mental health issues in patients visiting primary care physicians came to be called the de facto mental health system (Norquist & Regier, 1996). That graduating general physicians were ill-prepared to satisfy the psychosocial needs of their patients had long been of concern to medical educators, sociologists and some physicians (Smith, 2011; Smith et al., 2014). To compensate for this deficiency, since at least the 1960s and 1970s, individual psychiatrists, psychoanalysts and professional organizations offered training for their non-psychiatrist colleagues through lectures, seminars, symposia, books and, more recently, computerized continuing medical education (CME) courses; results have been questionable, at times null. In England during the 1950s and 1960s, Michael Balint embarked on an endeavor to address this problem with a very different approach. The above quotation by a Balint Group participant is a limited view of Balint's own perspective on his work, although it does reflect the attitude of some of the early recruits to Balint Groups.

This chapter will focus on Michael Balint's seminal psychoanalytic work on applying innovative ways of bringing fuller understanding of patients and their physicians through the application of "overall diagnosis," contrasted with the more limited typical physician focus on "objective illness." We include a brief account of Balint's early life, his career journey, roots of his group work with physicians, the nature of and impact of "Balint Groups" on both leader and participants, as well as his place in the psychoanalytic milieu of his time, with special reference to his unique relationship with Sandor Ferenczi.

DOI: 10.4324/9781003167679-12

A Word about Psychoanalysis Applied to Medicine

Psychoanalysis was conceived and delivered in a matrix of medicine by a physician. Nonetheless, their continuing relationship had a well-documented vacillating and often tentative kinship (Lipsitt, 2020). Freud noted early in his career that a great deal of counseling and likely personal growth occurred in the offices of general physicians the world over, although psychoanalysis nonetheless remained virtually unknown as a resource to both physicians and their patients in general practice. Freud had hoped to find a way to enhance the "psychotherapeutic function" of general medical practice with application of newly discovered psychoanalytic knowledge.

In an address delivered before the 5th International Psycho-analytic Congress in Budapest in 1918, he had predicted that "at some time or other the conscience of the community will awake and admonish it that the poor man has just as much right to help for his mind as he now has to the surgeon's means of saving life … In other words, ways would be found to help those with emotional suffering as much as with organic illnesses" (Freud, 1919, p. 167). He stated further that "the task will then arise for us to adapt our techniques to the new conditions" (ibid., p. 168). He did not disparage or rule out "active" approaches to achieve this result, contrary to the perception of some later biographers. He acknowledged that "It is very probable … that the application of our therapy to numbers will compel us to alloy the pure gold of analysis plentifully with the copper of direct suggestion" (ibid.). He concluded his remarks with the prediction that "whatever form this psychotherapy for the people may take, whatever the elements out of which it is compounded, its most effective and most important ingredients, will assuredly remain those borrowed from strict psycho-analysis, which serves no ulterior purpose" (ibid.). There is no doubt that Michael Balint, still a medical student in 1918, heard and was moved by Freud's address!

Despite Freud's impassioned wish to see psychoanalysis applied to common medical practice, his touch-and-go relationship with medicine redirected his interest to other pursuits (Lipsitt, 2020). Freud abandoned attempts in the Project for a Scientific Psychology (originally called a Psychology for Neurologists) to create Helmholtzian theories to explain the symptoms of the hysterical patients in his medical practice through physiological and neurological concepts. He essentially left it to others to explore how psychoanalysis might have application to other fields. This notion of applied psychoanalysis has most commonly been associated with aspects of art, history, literature, anthropology and philosophy. Freud himself was known, in his writings, to apply the principles of psychoanalysis to subjects such as Moses, Leonardo da Vinci and Hamlet, but not medicine.

Freud's enduring tentativeness to pair psychoanalysis with medicine is undoubtedly multidetermined; for many decades it has been argued that analysis has (or hasn't) been a part of medicine per se. Freud ultimately asserted that, in fact, a medical degree was a non-essential requisite for psychoanalytic training and practice (Freud, 1925, 1926). It would remain for psychoanalysts like Michael Balint, in the third "watershed," to fulfill Freud's early wishes and prediction. Relevant to this advancement, a member of the French Balint Society (Gendrot, 1972) wrote that "for 30 years, from 1926 to 1956, an enormous gulf appeared between medicine and psychoanalysis, and the deep misunderstandings that resulted were prejudiced to both disciplines." Medicine was becoming more objective, measurable and physically observable (antibiotics, X-rays, surgical approaches). Psychoanalysis became more focused on theories and treatments for subjective woes (trauma, conflicts, troubles in work and love).

> Until the appearance of Balint ... [in the 1950s], the efforts of doctors and psychoanalysts who were trying to come together and understand each other, were rendered futile by a total lack of knowledge ... Balint [was able] to distinguish between medicine and psychoanalysis, as well as providing a method of initiating a dialogue between them, to the advantage of both.
>
> (Gendrot, 1972, p. 300)

Freud discovered the "talking cure" by helping his friend Breuer contend with his patient, Anna O., who had distressingly fallen in love with him to the point that she hallucinated she was carrying his child. The hysterics of Vienna (like the patients Freud had observed in Charcot's clinic in Paris) provided the first group of symptomatic patients for whom psychoanalysis provided effective treatment. Letting her tell her story, her "chimney sweeping" as she called it (Breuer & Freud, 1895, p. 30) allowed her to discover in Freud's presence that her thoughts were not reality but fantasies and strong desires that could dissolve in speaking to a carefully listening doctor. This epochal moment became the beginning of free association, psychoanalysis and a process that would be expanded on by Balint and others in acknowledging the primacy of the patient.

The Contributions of Michael Balint in the Third Watershed

The Early Years

It appears that, in some sense, Balint was destined to ally himself with medicine, whatever turns his life may take in the journey (Engel, 2020). Interest abounds as to how Balint became so committed to applying his psychoanalytic knowledge and skills to helping general practitioners be more attentive to the psychosocial aspects of their work (Paulsen, 2019). In a revealing interview (Hopkins, 1972, p. 317ff.) one month before his death, Balint responded promptly to this question: "First, my father was a general practitioner for about 50 years in Budapest until his death, so I grew up in this atmosphere ... [After graduation] I had to stand in for my father and so I had some understanding of what general practice was" (ibid., p. 317). In what may perhaps be a kind of pre-death insight, Balint said "But all this was not really known by me consciously; it was there" (ibid.). This awareness will become clearer as we trace Balint's career and gravitation toward group work with general practitioners.

From early on, young Balint was a kind of existential experimentalist. He flirted with engineering, physics and chemistry before pursuing a medical education, urged on him by his father. In fact, his interview with Hopkins revealed that "I almost became an electrical engineer; it was really touch and go" (Hopkins, 1972, p. 317). Like Freud, he found courses in philosophy, comparative law and religion, and anthropology more appealing than the standard curriculum, all the while maintaining his curiosity about physics and chemistry. Interrupted by the war, he graduated medical school in 1920 at age 24, intending to pursue his early interest in biochemistry.

During his early years in Budapest, Michael's interest in psychoanalysis had been catalyzed by Freud's Totem and Tattoo (Freud, 1913), gifted to him by girlfriend Alice Szekely-Kovacs, the woman who would become his wife; she was a classmate of Michael's sister Emma and the daughter of a Hungarian training analyst Vilma Kovacs. Married shortly after medical graduation, he and Alice left Hungary for Berlin, a city rich scientifically and culturally. It is unclear whether this questionably precipitous move to Berlin so soon after medical graduation and marriage was in some way related to family tension and dynamics. Michael and his father allegedly did not get along well, with father described as authoritarian, aggressive and punitive (Swerdloff, 2002; Moreau-Ricaud, 2015); one biographer (Moreau-Ricaud, 2015, p. 173) also claims that young Michael, although "...a very clever pupil with an enormous curiosity... nevertheless could be a scamp and make mischief, [and] as an adolescent, to regularly challenge his father," reputedly a well-regarded general physician.

Although the title "revolutionary" is commonly assigned to pioneering Hungarians, perhaps this appellation was attached to Michael from an early age, when he was also labeled (and later proudly accepted) the moniker of enfant terrible (Oppenheim-Gluckman, 2015; Moreau-Ricaud, 2015; Engel, 2020).

At some point, Michael had changed his name from Mihaly Bergsmann to Michael Balint and abandoned his Jewish heritage for Unitarianism, an event of great disappointment and unhappiness to his orthodox parents. The exact date of this name change is fuzzy, although one biographer dates it to late adolescence, age 17 (Swerdloff, 2002), well before Nazism seemed a likely precipitant (coincidentally, Ferenczi's father had also changed the family name from Fraenkel). Allegedly, strained relations between father and son persisted until after Michael's later emigration with Alice to Manchester,

England in 1939. The estrangement, in the face of oncoming Nazi threats at that time, may have significantly impelled Michael to seek reconciliation with his father. Alice had died from a ruptured aneurysm 6 months after their move to Manchester, a great emotional trauma to Balint, leaving him with a young son.

The compounded losses of both wife and parents undoubtedly affected Michael's path forward; an attempt at re-marriage in 1944, perhaps to secure a mother for his son and a new companion for himself, faltered soon after but without divorce until 1952 during his time at Tavistock Clinic. There he would meet and marry Enid Eichholz in 1958, his new collaborator in group studies. According to grown son John Balint (personal communication), who had become a gastroenterologist and ethics professor in the United States, there was eventual reconciliation with his father, but only just before Michael's parents, remaining in Hungary, in 1944 (same year he entered the ill-fated marriage) took their own lives by cyanide poisoning to avoid arrest by Nazis.

A Serendipitous Career

One's career path seldom reflects a unilateral trajectory toward its final goal. Most usually zig-zag, with many digressions toward a final objective. Very often, it is a concatenation of randomly experienced events that eventually determine an individual's career commitment. Such was the experience of Michael Balint; Balint's entry into his famed explorations with physician groups took a number of serendipitous turns. The work for which he is best known emerged only late in his career in the 1950s and flourished until obligatory (UK) retirement from Tavistock at age 65 (Gosling, 1966). Thus, the corpus of his group studies spanned little more than a decade!

Whether Michael had some clear objective in mind to pursue further study in biochemistry or was eager to flee the tumultuous relationship with his practitioner father is unclear; it was still early to be threatened by the Nazi invasion of Europe. Nevertheless, in Berlin, Michael seemed to nurture continuing thoughts of a career in biochemistry, finding work in a biochemistry lab with a future Nobel Prize laureate, Otto Warburg, while simultaneously pursuing a doctorate in biochemistry (historical notes are not persuasive that he had been actually invited to that position), receiving his PhD in biochemistry, physics and biology; later, with an interest in childhood development, he would also complete requirements for the MSc degree in genetic psychology (Balint, 1966, pp. 125–162).

Alice continued her pursuits in anthropology and ethnology. Although Michael felt his main interest continued in physics and chemistry, he and Alice retained their mutual intrigue with psychoanalysis by beginning personal analyses with Hans Sachs; disappointed in Sachs's didacticism (and arguably his lack of medical training, perhaps of relevance in his subsequent analysis with Ferenczi), they terminated with Sachs.

According to Balint (Hopkins, 1972, p. 316), during his years in Berlin, he also became interested in psychosomatic medicine (Freud's disciples, especially Felix Deutsch, had begun in those years to publish in that domain) and published early papers on that subject (although not listed in his bibliography). A description of Balint's life and work (Oppenheim-Gluckman, 2015) suggests that he published an article in 1923 (Balint, 1923) on the role of psychoanalysis in the service of general practitioners during this period (but this paper cannot be found). In Europe, he was engaged in jobs essentially unrelated to either psychoanalysis or later group work: a directorship of a Child Guidance Clinic; the Institute of Organic Chemistry of the Royal Academy of Berlin; physician in Charite Hospital medical clinic; and unspecified various positions in the Psychoanalytic Institute, headed by Karl Abraham.

On return to Budapest just a few years later, in 1924, he first worked as an assistant in the Medical Institute of the University Medical Clinic and entered analysis with Sandor Ferenczi, an event that may have had significant impact on crystallizing firmer career directions (*vide infra*). While still a medical student, he had already been familiar with Freud's 1918 lecture and impressed by Ferenczi's 1919 lectures to general physicians; he later appreciated a lecture by Ferenczi to the Kassa Hungarian Physicians' Society emphasizing the notion that psychoanalysis should play an important role in everyday life (Oppenheim-Gluckman, 2015, p. 65). When he began as a member of the Hungarian Psychoanalytic Institute, he noted a wish of the institute to "get more doctors interested in psychoanalysis." In an interview, he recalled that "I was asked to run seminars for general practitioners on exactly the same sort of psychological understanding [as psychoanalysis]" (Hopkins, 1972, p. 319). On the request of local doctors in a provincial town in Hungary, he gave a lecture on psychological problems in medicine (Balint, 1926). "The intention was above all to raise awareness among GPs by way of theoretical instruction" (Oppenheim-Gluckmann, 2015, p. 66).

Freud had hoped to make Budapest a kind of capital of psychoanalysis, appointing Ferenczi president of an International Psychoanalytic Society there, but these plans dissolved in the wake of political unrest in the wake of war. Balint reported that such activity was interfered with by local police and had to be abandoned in 1936 until he could resume such activity in England (Hopkins, 1972, 318). These experiences demonstrate Balint's life-long interest in working with general practitioners.

In 1924, with 23 years between them, Balint's analyst Sandor Ferenczi appointed him deputy assistant in the latter's recently opened Polyclinic for the integrated treatment of impecunious patients (Ferenczi was the first University Professor of Psychoanalysis). In 1926, Balint had become a member of the nascent Hungarian Psychoanalytic Society, joining Ferenczi in the formation of the second Psychoanalytic Society, following Freud's Institute in Vienna. The Hungarian institute adopted Ferenczi's practice of the analysand's psychoanalyst also being his or her first supervisor, an arrangement that speaks to developmental concepts deeply embedded in both Ferenczi's and Balint's notion of psychoanalytic training. The analyst was the shepherd, or the Sherpa, of the candidate's growth. The patient's wisdom was innate, defenses and even character problems such as narcissism (which Balint explicated in his book *The Basic Fault*, describing a deficit in loving; Balint, 1968) could be brought into mutual attention, questioning and healing.

On Ferenczi's death in 1933, Balint became Director of the Clinic and the Budapest Psychoanalytic Institute. The unusual relationship between analysand and colleague of Ferenczi cannot escape closer examination for the influence of Ferenczi on Balint's career as well as his theories and clinical methods (Freud, 1924).

The Ferenczi Connection

Balint's relationship with Ferenczi became an unusually intense one and of formative importance in Balint's subsequent endeavors. Atypical of relationships between analysts and their analysands, Balint not only became a friend, translator of much of Ferenczi's literary work (Ferenczi, 1980a, 1980b, 1984), but also his obituarist (Balint, 1933a) and estate executive; they wrote occasional papers together (Dimitrijevic et al, 2018; Moreau-Ricaud, 2015). Balint was said to have been familiar with a book by Ferenczi and Rank on the development of psychoanalysis (Ferenczi & Rank, 1923). Balint's chapter on "The Unobtrusive Analyst" in his book *The Basic Fault* (Balint, 1968, pp. 173–181) emphasized the need of the analyst to "let the patient be himself," a precursor of similar to later remarks by Winnicott:

> The analyst lets the patient set the pace and he does the next best thing to letting the patient decide when to come and go… [the analyst] seeking his way among the mass of material offered and trying to find out what, at the moment, is the shape and form of the thing which he has to offer the patient.
> (Winnicott, 1984, pp. 52–69)

Ferenczi had also emphasized that:

> the patient should be able to find himself, to accept himself, and to get on with himself … moreover, he must be allowed to discover his way to the world of objects and not be shown the 'right' way by some profound or correct interpretation.
> (Oppenheim-Gluckman, 2015, p. 14)

This principle would later become a prominent hallmark of Balint Groups. Ferenczi had so strongly advocated for the participation of psychoanalysts in medical care that, as early as 1923, he introduced the revolutionary idea that sanatoriums caring for patients with pulmonary disease should compulsorily include a psychoanalyst as part of the medical team (ibid., p. 17).

Balint followed Ferenczi, as noted, in giving early lectures to general practitioners in Budapest in the early 1920s. Much of Balint's approach to working with general practitioners had filtered down and been absorbed from ideas shared with his analyst. Intense interest in the nuanced interactions between patient and physician was at the core of both their attitudes toward medical (and psychoanalytic) care. Balint had also subscribed to Ferenczi's ideas of the importance of the "atmosphere of the analytic situation or consultation" (ibid., p. 6) and the importance of the mother-child relationship or "maternal care" in "overcoming resistances" (ibid., p. 6), not dissimilar to Winnicott's "holding environment" (Winnicott, 1963, p. 74).

Those inclined to take a psychoanalytic approach to Balint's relationship with Ferenczi will not find it difficult to recognize the father transference to his analyst. In an obituary by Balint on Ferenczi's death, he had written in adulatory tones of the "loss of our movement" (Balint, 1933a). Balint became Ferenczi's literary executor and was responsible for posthumous publication of much of the latter's writings (Ferenczi, 1980a, 1980b, 1984). "Ferenczi's inheritance had profoundly influenced Balint's clinical practice and theories" (Oppenheim-Gluckman, 2015, p. 20).

An intriguing triumvirate developed among Balint, Ferenczi and Georg Groddeck. Mutual friendships with George Groddeck, a physician and self-styled psychoanalyst who had attracted Freud's interest (Freud, 1924), had stimulated curiosity in "psychosomatic illness." Groddeck and Balint both undervalued "traditional" medical practice, the former establishing a sanitarium where he provided a mixture of classical and nontraditional methods like diet, hydrotherapy and massage (he did not believe in drugs), and the latter referring to the "apostolic function" adhered to by physicians who slavishly practiced only "objective" medicine. Balint, Ferenczi and Groddeck had all been practicing physicians, with fathers who were also general physicians.

It was like "family." Curiously, Ferenczi, on recommendation of Felix Deutsch in 1921, sought medical treatment for pyelonephritis from Groddeck at his Baden-Baden sanatorium, and even brought his family there both for treatment and holiday. Later, Ferenczi took Groddeck as an analysand. Balint and Ferenczi shared correspondence with Groddeck over the meaning of the "It" and its resemblance to Freud's "id." Freud, the "strict constructionist," was nevertheless enthralled with Groddeck, his behavior and his ideas until finally severing relations. Like Balint, Groddeck felt "treatment was based on the idea that the doctor was merely the catalyst who starts off the therapeutic process." At age 64, Groddeck wrote, "I am as aware as Freud that psychoanalysis is a world-wide affair and only partly a medical affair and that its tie-up with medicine is a disaster" (Schacht, 1977, p. 1).

Groddeck, Ferenczi and Balint were all at various times thought of in psychoanalytic circles as a bit marginal in their ideas (Rachman, 1999), with both Ferenczi and Balint referred to variously in biographical literature as "enfants terrible" (Engel, 2020; Swerdloff, 2002). All challenged Freud's established tenets of psychoanalysis in evolving their own concepts. For sure, the kind of practice engaged in by Michael Balint was quite out of the mainstream of practicing psychoanalysts of his time; he often referred to himself as an "outsider." From a current-day perspective, important elements of both Ferenczi and Balint's ideas are no longer "outside" the mainstream of psychoanalytic practice.

The importance of Balint's relationship to Ferenczi in the light of Balint's later work cannot be minimized. He would make liberal use of concepts of free association, transference and countertransference, regression, symptom formation, repression and the like, espoused by Ferenczi in his later group activity with physicians. Balint's perspective on the requisite skills of the general practitioner came not only from his younger days when he made rounds with his general practitioner father and from his lectures to general practitioners in Budapest, but also from his strong affiliation with Ferenczi (Balint, 1933b, 1948, 1958). Even after becoming a psychoanalyst, he never lost sight of the necessity for all physicians to be comfortably skilled in addressing his or her patients' accompanying emotional response to virtually all disease. He maintained interest in studying and helping non-psychiatrists and non-psychoanalysts serve their patients to their fullest ability.

The lineage from Freud to Ferenczi to Balint is prominent (Moreau-Ricaud, 2015). In this regard, both Balint and Ferenczi strayed little from Freud's own words in a 1904 lecture to a group of practicing Viennese physicians:

> psychotherapy is in no way a modern method of treatment ... it is the most ancient form of therapy in medicine ... psychotherapeutic endeavors of one kind or another have never completely disappeared from medicine ... We physicians cannot discard psychotherapy, if only because another person intimately concerned in the process of recovery – the patient – has no intention of discarding it ... All physicians, yourselves included, are constantly practicing psychotherapy, even when you have no intention of doing so and are not aware of it; it is a disadvantage, however, to leave the mental factor in your treatment so completely in the patient's hands. Thus, it is impossible to keep a check on it, to administer it in doses or to intensify it. Is it not then a justifiable endeavor on the part of the physician to seek to obtain command of this factor, to use it with a purpose, and to direct and strengthen it? This and nothing else is what scientific psychotherapy proposes.
>
> (Freud, 1904)

"These diseases (psychoneuroses) are not cured by the drug but by the physician, that is by the personality of the physician, inasmuch as through it he exerts a mental influence" (ibid., p. 251). Were these comments an incubus for Balint's, as well as Ferenczi's, common practice with groups to speak of the "drug doctor"? We can notice in this early statement that the emphasis is on the "personality of the physician," rather than the relationship between the patient and physician. Ferenczi had also written of ways in which "the doctor prescribes himself" as well as how the "physician responds to the patient's offerings," ideas that became part of Balint's group lexicon (Balint, 1957a, 1957b; Lacan, 2001).

Ferenczi likewise had written "the Faculty does not tell us how to dose this medication, nor what are its modes of actions, while psychoanalysis provides precise knowledge and well-defined methods on this question" (Oppenheim-Gluckman, 2015). These comments might very well have been appropriated by Balint as the gateway to helping physicians develop more self-understanding that, in turn, helped them to better care for the relationships with their patients. The reference to the physician as "drug" was fully explicated in Balint's book, *The Doctor, the Patient and the Illness* (Balint, 1957a), while it is of curious interest that the book does not mention either Ferenczi or Freud; it does, however, refer frequently to psychoanalysis. Nonetheless, there is an echo of Freud when Balint writes:

> pure gold has the remarkable quality of withstanding any fire and even being purified by it. I do not see any reason why we should be afraid for the essential parts of our science, and should any of its minor frills burn away, being not of pure gold, the better for future generations.
> (Balint, 1968, p. 103)

In 1939, Michael at the age of 42 gave up his directorship of the Budapest Psychoanalytic Institute and with Alice emigrated to Manchester (not London), invited by his friend John Rickman. Rickman had been President of the International Psychoanalytic Society at the time; both had been analyzed by Ferenczi (Rickman had also spent analytic time with Freud and Melanie Klein). There, from 1942 to 1945, Michael worked as a "psychiatric consultant" in the Manchester Northern Royal Hospital, teaching medicine and science, and did "a little analytic work." During those years, he was also director of Centers for Child Guidance in Northeast Lancaster and Preston (it is recalled that he had obtained a master's degree in child psychology!). In 1947 he became a British citizen and a member of the Tavistock Institute in 1948. In 1955, he was elected president of the medical section of the British Psychological Society (Oppenheim-Gluckman, 2015). By 1968 he was installed as president of the British Psychoanalytic Society, a position he held until his death in 1970 at age 74. Mandatory retirement required that he leave his post at the Tavistock Institute at age 65.

Although interest in working with and teaching general practitioners allegedly began with Michael in Budapest around 1924, it did not flourish until after he migrated to Britain in 1939. While working in Manchester, he was once more invited by John Rickman in 1945 at the age of 49 to visit the Tavistock Clinic as a consultant to a social worker and psychoanalyst, Enid Eichholz, who was working with families helping to improve their social adjustment. She had studied psychoanalysis with Rickman and helped to found the Family Discussion Bureau (1955) incorporated into the Tavistock Institute in the late 1940s for the purpose of providing supervision and training of social workers to deal with marital and family problems (Gosling, 1966); here he began observing the groups run by Enid. The Institute had already tried offering courses to general practitioners returning from military service, without much success. Balint was asked to join the program for social workers run by Enid, whom he married in 1958. As he continued working with the social worker groups, he began grafting his own approach on to that of sessions that were already being provided, an alliance in which, as Enid later wrote, Michael had all but "taken us over." He introduced the proposal that they not read from case reports but rather engage in a more free-associative way of discussing cases. Perhaps in observing the groups of social workers, Michael saw a paradigm of what would become The Balint Group. In family dynamics, the relationship between mothers and their babies is often the most important focus of family life. Winnicott by this time had already written that there is no such thing as a baby, or a mother, there is only a baby and a mother (Winnicott, 1963). For general practitioners and their patients, it would be the relationship between them that would be the central topic of the discussion in a Balint Group.

Balint also benefitted in understanding group dynamics through his association in the Clinic with Wilfred Bion (1961), who had been studying group dynamics for several years at Tavistock, soon giving it up to exclusively study psychotic individuals. Michael Balint began his first training-cum-research group at the Tavistock Clinic in 1950 and continued with this work until retirement at age 65. Nevertheless, he continued to speak, write and meet with aspiring Balint groups throughout the world. He also visited the University of Cincinnati annually as a visiting professor in applied psychoanalysis. There, he collaborated extensively with Doctors Paul and Anna Ornstein.

Beginnings of the "Balint Group"

As Balint began, with Enid, his research into physician–patient relations, he was able, through a newspaper notice, to attract several interested physicians (including psychiatrists) who wanted to capitalize on their war experience to improve their general practice. The post-war establishment of the National Health Service in 1946 meant that patients would have free access to physicians, imposing a greater burden on physicians and awareness of the need for greater psychological understanding of their patients. Also, Britain had pioneered in the concept of "patient-centered medicine" at the time. This concatenation of vectors provided a propitious setting for offering training. However, nothing was easy. Even with willing volunteers, Balint wrote that a number either soon dropped out or were unsuitable for the endeavor (Balint et al., 1966, p. 31). In time, the category of general practitioner (GP) evolved into specialists of all stripes or primary care physicians (also designated as a kind of specialty). Nonetheless, he made it his life work to help physicians achieve this "impossible" objective, trying to understand why "this collaborative work between psychoanalysts and doctors is so difficult, so problematic" (Balint et al., 1966, p. 26).

His work gradually was recognized and adapted around the world, first in France in 1967 with the French Balint Society, subsequently in Britain with the Balint Society in 1969, an International Balint Federation in 1972, and not until 1990, the American Balint Society (ABS), despite significant prior interest in the United States, where Balint was invited every 2 years to Cincinnati to teach his methods (Maurice Levine, chair of psychiatry at Cincinnati, wrote an introduction to Balint's 1957 book *The Doctor, His Patient and the Illness*, describing it as "an important event for the general practitioners and for the psychiatrists in this country [for whom] the time is ripe for serious consideration of fundamental research on the function and practice of the 'family doctor'"; Levine, 1957, p. v).

Rise of the Independents

In Britain, Balint seemed to have found a "home." Several prominent analysts, including such "independents" as Donald Winnicott, Ronald Fairbairn, John Bowlby, Wilfred Bion, Franz Alexander and others who elected to pursue rather nontraditional paths. Several of these British psychoanalysts commonly challenged Freud's postulates and became known as The British Independents. Balint was welcomed warmly to this group, with vital exchange of ideas among all. In some aspect of their psychoanalytic experience, all applied their knowledge of developmental psychology and analysis to areas of medical care, largely contributing to what became known as the object relations school of psychoanalytic theory; they generally subscribed to "two-person" therapeutic relations (akin to patient–physician relations) rather than the "one-person" Oedipal focus of orthodox Freudian psychoanalysis. Winnicott, well known for the expressions "the good mother" and "the holding environment" (Winnicott, 1963, p. 74) continued throughout his career to address both physical and emotional problems of children, while expressing the physician's vexing difficulty in "riding the two horses (psyche and soma)" (Winnicott, 1966). Fairbairn considered the "mutative factors in psychotherapy as the 'good relationship' between the therapist and patient" (Wikipedia, 2021). Bowlby, during the World War II, treated affected children in child guidance clinics; after the war, he became deputy director of

Tavistock Clinic and from 1950 mental health consultant to the World Health Organization.

Michael Balint, in studying the patient–physician relationships of general medical practice, perhaps took this trend further than most. More than others of the British Independent Group, he is best known for the legacy of his work with medical practitioners, later to be known as Balint Groups. In his 1966 article, Psychoanalysis and Medicine, Balint asks "Shall we analysts accept any responsibility in this field? Or shall we keep out of it?" He bolsters his own position by quoting Freud's prediction in 1918 "that the time would come when society must accept that the individual has the same right for help in his neurotic or emotional suffering as in his organic illnesses" (Balint, 1966, p. 54). Balint writes in the affirmative:

> in recent years, the training of general practitioners and nonpsychiatric specialties ... has become a public problem of some importance ... A substantial number of people asking for surgical and medical assistance are in fact suffering from emotional problems [as noted repeatedly by others]. To offer them surgical or medical treatment has proved inefficient and unhelpful, a waste of time, money and energy, and has often amounted to gross neglect or even cruelty.
> (Balint, 1966, p. 54)

Of some curiosity is that in writing, after legal retirement from Tavistock, *The Crisis of Medical Practice* (Balint, 2002), Balint had listed his only title as PhD (not MD), perhaps intending to reclaim his background in science applied to his later work in psychoanalysis and medicine!

It was the convergence of a perfect storm of natural events following World War II in England that created the conditions for a sea change in the collaboration between psychoanalysis and general practice. Many of Europe's psychoanalytic pioneers, Freud and Balint among them, had fled Hitler to take refuge in England. The post-war healthcare system in England recognized that a great burden of everyday mental suffering was falling in the laps of general practitioners. It was also a time when hospitals were beginning to develop departments of Family Medicine (Player et al., 2018). The Tavistock Clinic and Institute provided a center where many of Freud's followers installed an effective system of helping mothers and childcare workers through a group process including observation, discussion and experience-based learning. On a personal level, Michael Balint was contending with the memory of his parents' refusal to flee Hungary, committing suicide to avoid capture by the SS.

Wilfred Bion (1961), known for his studies of group dynamics, contributing heavily to the interest in groups at the Tavistock Institute. Alexander, considered by many as an early contributor to the field of psychosomatic medicine, coined the expression "corrective emotional experience"

(Alexander, 1950; Alexander & French, 1946). Ferenczi challenged many of Freud's postulates, preferring a more active (than passive) approach to therapy, focused largely on regression and transference/countertransference issues in their relevance to all forms of patient–doctor relationship issues (Ferenczi, 1923, 1982). Perhaps more than others, he persisted in trying to find ways to shorten analytic treatment to make it more applicable to a larger number of patients with varieties of ailments and to promote their usefulness to the wider field of general medicine. This new direction provided the latticework for Balint's own development of "focal" psychotherapy, as well as that of Malan (1963), Sifneos, Mann, Davanloo and others who later developed short-term treatment methods. Balint's innovations in this direction are described in a book on the topic as "an example of applied psychoanalysis" (Balint et al., 1972).

Balint saw the possible creative collaboration resulting from an amalgam of various vectors provided him at the Tavistock. He approached the British healthcare system to create a program that would allow general practitioners to attend Tavistock-like groups fortnightly. These groups, led by Michael and Enid Balint, would provide an active mutual learning environment to facilitate professional growth, enhanced capacity to handle the personal demands from their patients, and to bolster their own personal resilience in their practice. Although increasingly quite popular, it was not always easy to assemble and lead early groups, requiring Balint to train others in his method of group leadership. His wife, Enid, became active in directing and studying the particular qualities of profession-based groups. Balint recorded much of this early work in his book, *The Doctor, His Patient, and the Illness* (Balint, 1957a).

Perhaps of some moment, several of these independent psychoanalysts were born into families of physician fathers, including Ferenczi and Balint. And most had served as physicians during World War II, some offering service to soldiers with war trauma. From their psychoanalytic training and experience, further recognition of issues related to transference and countertransference figured prominently in their work. All shared an interest with Ferenczi in finding ways to shorten the course of psychoanalysis to make it applicable to a larger number of patients with varieties of ailments. In later decades, analysts like Grete Bibring and others (Bibring, 1956; Kahana & Bibring, 1956), trained in classical psychoanalysis, innovated ways to make psychoanalytic precepts useful to medical practice in general hospital medical-surgical services.

A Bridge Between Psychoanalysis and General Practice

Like many forms of practice or discipline that nourish the practitioners of the healing arts, the Balint Group, as mentioned, with derivatives from many sources, had its origins largely in the biography of one man, his narrative, and the way his own journey came to be applied to a purpose. The purpose often resolves a conflict like that of the Hero Myth; the hero begins with a wound, then journeys to find a way to both heal the wound, and to see if his own discovery can provide healing powers to suffering of the larger world.

The "Balint Group"

The centrality of a Balint group, as it emerged, is its focus on the relationship between doctor and patient. The details of the patient's illness and background facts are briefly described and the group has a chance to ask "clarifying questions" for a short period of time following the presenter's description of his case. The case may be: "What about this patient who keeps me up at night?" "What about this patient who makes my heart sink when I see her on my schedule in the morning?" The patients are not in the room, as babies were with their mothers in Enid's mother–infant groups, but focused on the relationship dilemmas, to bring the patient–doctor relationship into the room, so to speak, like a two-person hologram that comes alive in the imaginations of the group members. After the case is described and factual questions asked, the group leaders invite the presenter to "push back" from the group, in a literal moving of the chair back a bit. This ritual is particularly true of Balint groups as practiced in the USA. Although the American Balint Society acknowledges that in Europe, South America and elsewhere in the world, Balint groups may have the presenter remain "in" the group. The "pushback" in American Balint groups is a small formal ritual that reinforces that the presenter is no longer an active participant in the next phase of the group's work. This physical formality makes the statement that the presenter now cannot be directly addressed by the rest of the group, cannot be asked questions, and literally sits in a space where she/he is allowed to simply listen to the group work and to muse on his/her own thoughts.

The next phase of the group's work comes to resemble quite profoundly the theoretical notions of relational psychoanalysis and field theory. These groups form a bridge between psychoanalysis and general practice. Psychoanalysis can seem very complex, arcane, at one end and at the other end intuitively true, based in common sense. Freud's early ambition at the turn of the last century was to create a new neuro-psychiatric treatment within the accepted heart of traditional medicine. His explorations of early childhood, instinctual drives of sex and aggression, the influence of past patterns on present behavior, became a revolutionary understanding of man's inner life on a par with Darwin's theories about the biological origins of our species. Clinically, he demonstrated the power of a skilled transformative relationship to remove symptoms, facilitate behavior change, and improve work and interpersonal life. Despite these innovative achievements, for the first half of the 20th century, Freud's realm of psychoanalysis existed outside the body of medicine.

There are several basic components that distinguish a Balint Group.

1 The case.
2 The process.
3 The results.

Since its inception, a Balint group almost always begins with the question, "who has a case?" The usual size of a group is 7–10 members with a facilitator. If the group meets every other week, and takes the summer off, that will mean that each member has two or three cases to present in the course of a year. "A case" is most often a patient relationship which has created a feeling of conflict, being stuck or being lost in the physician. Other sources of case material that have worked well have included interactions with hospital or clinic administration, relationships with professional colleagues, trainees, supervisors, partners, and so on. The manner of presentation is that of a "curbside consultation." The work of the group facilitator is to assure two elements:

1 specificity of detail, encouraging the presenter to shy away from generalizations, to bring a detailed and associatively gathered description of the event (here we see the principle of free association, borrowed from psychoanalysis, applied to the Balint process), or course of interaction; and
2 that the dilemma, or "bother," felt by the clinician in the case is included in the presentation, particularly as the presentation draws to a close and the discussion is about to be handed over to the group.

The focus on the dilemma is enabled by questions like, "What troubled you about that?" or "What threw you off your stride at that point?" From a psychoanalytic point of view questions like "what troubled you" are at the edge of ego function – that perimeter of self-encountering experience that registers whether something is amiss. It bears fruit in a Balint process because it fits with the effort of the presenter to bring in experience of the case that is not pre-digested, that includes affective coloring from the physician's encounter without making the emotional self a focus of the interaction.

This point is very important to emphasize because many a Balint group has been rejected by a physician who felt in the question "how did you feel about that?" that professional growth has just been turned into pseudo-psychotherapy. It is another basic principle from psychoanalysis that if you ask for feelings, one is much more likely to get resistance to participation. The feelings are indeed present or the doctor would not be troubled by the experience. However, they are permitted to come out naturally, to be recognized either by the group or the physician herself, in the wake of carefully described specific details of the case. It was one of Balint's most extraordinary talents to be able to convey psychoanalytic concepts in their simplest, most jargon-free, everyday language.

In describing the process of a Balint group it is as important to describe what it is not. It is not the application of psychoanalytic formulations to patient/physician dilemmas. It is not psychotherapy. The facilitator is not the expert, but rather joins with the group of physicians in discovering what needs to be understood about the case. The stance and prospect of mutual discovery is what makes a Balint group an accepted and sought-after collaboration between doctors and analysts. The focus is on self-discovery, not on self-disclosure. It reminds the analyst that while her skills may be helpful to this process of discovery, it is not her knowledge of human development, conflict, defense or any other psychoanalytic theory that provides the useful grist for the doctors' mill.

The physician is the fundamental authority when it comes to her experience, but the magic of the Balint group happens as the doctor tells her story to the group. Two things start to happen simultaneously: first, she is talking to a group of peers and does not have to tailor what she is saying, allowing for a kind of contained free association to occur as she talks, and she finds herself saying things she didn't know she knew, feeling things she didn't know she felt; secondly, the group of listening doctors are putting themselves in her shoes, finding congruencies and incongruencies, imagining their own recent or remote experiences with similar patients or circumstances. The densely packed experience of the presenter becomes unpacked, arrayed in the room. It can almost seem that the doctor's experience is becoming visible to herself. The group then can take up these unpacked descriptions and try them on as in "I had a patient somewhat like that" or "As I was listening to you, I wondered how I would have approached my colleague with that information." or "I had a similar experience with a family member dressing me down at a funeral."

This general discussion often leads to a discovery of some layers of feeling and experience in the presenter, the discovery of anger, feeling put down by the patient, complex feelings around accepting a gift, a sense of personal space being invaded by a patient. It also, at least in some groups, can lead to a plan of action: How is the doctor going to approach his next encounter with the patient? What possible diagnoses had not yet been considered? In the presenter-focused style of Balint process, in addition to keeping the presentation focused on specific details, the facilitator may make comments about the "shape" of the group process in response to the case. The nature of a group's response to a case, for example, of a malingering patient may be very different from the group discussion of a somatizing patient who turns out to have an occult malignancy. This kind of comparative, or linking, commentary can invigorate a group's awareness of how one dilemma will make itself felt differently from another, highlighting that the group process itself bears watching, that it has a liveliness and a specificity of its own.

Reflections from Balint Group members

What does a Balint group do for its members? One member stated it this way:

> In the first place, the sharing of a common experience, including particular difficulties we all encounter in patient care, is usually empowering. Also, the times when I am experiencing the most difficulty with a patient are usually associated with a feeling that I have become unmoored & entirely lost my direction.

Another member described his experience:

> Discussing the specifics of this situation with the group, even if it doesn't lead to concrete suggestions, often serves as a potent reality test and brings me back to earth. It allows me to return to the patient with a greater sense of confidence & direction.

The nature of this transformation from "unmoored and entirely losing a sense of direction" to being brought "back to earth" is at the heart of the Balint group's value. The transition from "lost" to "found" occurs in the process of presentation and discussion of the case among peers. Sometimes what is found are some hidden feelings, or what is lost is the clarity of purpose that the doctor needs to proceed with her work, to accomplish something in the visit, to make a plan for the next visit. Strangely, in the middle of a problematic case, vital perspective can be lost.

A primary care physician describes her experience of the Balint group in this way:

> The most obvious is the opportunity to discuss difficult cases ... sometimes difficult because of our reactions, sometime because of patient behavior, sometimes because of systemic problems that seem overwhelming. I have a sense of being out of balance in my thinking/judgment; but noticeably struggling inside where no one knows but me. Or I have had a series of cases or even one intense case. Emotions arise and I have no context in which I can process them. Most friends cannot understand the nuances of the medical setting unless you've done work there.

One wonderful example occurred when a group member, Dr. C, was describing his work with the spouse of his patient, Mr. M. Dr. C had cared for the couple for many years. The husband had succumbed to a cancer; the physician had attended his funeral, and a few months later the wife came in for her semi-annual physical. Ms. M. seemed depressed and related that she had tried talking to a psychiatrist whom a friend had recommended. She had given this up after a few sessions because she felt uneasy talking to a stranger. She began to cry and said in many ways that she would rather talk to Dr. C about the grief of missing her husband of forty years, since her physician had known him. Dr. C asked her to let him think about it and they would talk soon, scheduling a follow-up visit in a couple of weeks. Dr. C, an experienced internist, had always been interested in counseling and approached a senior psychoanalyst friend to see if he would supervise him doing a course of bereavement therapy with Ms. M. The analyst agreed. Ms. M. returned for her follow-up.

Dr. C and she embarked on 6 months of meeting every other week in bereavement therapy, which seemed to go very well, ending with Ms. M. tearfully thanking him for listening as they wound down for what they had decided would be their last therapy session. A few months later, Dr. C presented the case in a Balint group because he had found himself getting anxious about Ms. M's upcoming medical visit, her semi-annual physical. During the case presentation and subsequent group discussion, he realized that the focus of their relationship had changed during the therapy, that the conversational, physical ease they had shared over many years had now become a much more involved psychological closeness. Their relationship could not contain both types of closeness. At their next visit, he was able to describe his discovery to Ms. M., who expressed her own relieved anxiety. He found her a new internist. What had been a nameless anxiety became understood as a signal experience of the changing nature of boundaries in a close professional relationship.

Thus, the Balint Group provides a thoughtful perspective and a trusted environment where "my colleagues can hold my emotions with me." Similar experiences are shared by the Group. Finally, when all is said and done for a night's meeting, presented cases are referred to and asked about in subsequent meetings, allowing the group to learn from the case, the effectiveness [or not] of the group process and the ongoing experience of the presenter. It also serves as a place to discuss (both formally and informally) less difficult issues to work through possible approaches (we've discussed data and social issues around screening tests, for instance, though usually sparked by a particular case). As one member expressed:

> In addition, I value the support we give each other, as well as the challenge to rethink some patterns we might be stuck in ... There is both support and friendly confrontation that really helps me see more clearly and improve my care. Sometimes, it seems like the only place we really talk to each other about patients in a pure way, as our practice lives have become so much busier.

It is certainly true that not all cases presented in a Balint group have emotional complexity. Apparently, Michael Balint once implored one of his groups, "could somebody please present a case of a patient with a cold?"

Sometimes a seemingly simple case will lead to an exchange of information about practice styles. Two members of our Balint group discovered that they tended to see patients at a very different pace. They made a plan to visit one another's practice settings, spending several hours shadowing each other and in the next meeting talking about what they had observed in both practices.

From Bridge to Arc: Facilitators of the Boston Balint Group

The bridge between psychoanalysis and Balint Groups has undergone an evolutionary process in the last 30 years, with changes perhaps well illustrated through the arc of three successive facilitators of the Boston Balint Group. A brief description (from RHP) may give some personal perspective to this evolutionary view.

In roughly the period 1970 to 1985 psychoanalysis (particularly American) was evolving out of its dark period of strict adherence to anonymity, concern about "parameters" and rigid ideas of neutrality. In our experience with the Boston Balint group, these stages could be seen to operate in observable ways. One of the many unique aspects of the Boston Balint group is that it is has three long-term facilitators. Initially, Don Lipsitt was the invited facilitator from 1970. From 1985 to 2004, Randy Paulsen facilitated the group, after whom Eran Metzger, a psychiatrist certified by the ABS as a fully qualified Balint leader, faculty member and trainer, fulfilled the role from 2004 to the present.

Both Doctors Lipsitt and Paulsen are graduates of the Boston Psychoanalytic Society and Institute. Doctor Metzger has been trained in psychoanalytic psychotherapy and psychodynamic group therapy. All three have stood on separate but contiguous sections of the conceptual bridge between psychoanalysis and Balint groups.

Doctor Lipsitt began facilitating the Balint Group after several group members had attended a three-day intensive group workshop involving Balint-type sharing of case material. They recruited Lipsitt and several other interested general internists and primary care providers (a full description of this experience is in Lipsitt's 1998 paper on the Boston Balint group). DRL had edited occasional writings of Michael Balint, devoting an issue of his journal to Balint's work (Balint, 1970, p. 1) and was quite familiar with the basic ideas of a Balint group. Lipsitt's analytic training had largely been "classical," and he naturally brought that with him to the group as it began to meet on a bi-weekly basis.

Four examples come to mind from this period. In one group meeting, a member talked about the experience of receiving a beautiful gift from a patient. The discussion centered around other members having received gifts, both large and small, and that they tended to be viewed as gestures of gratitude, recognition and were universally accepted as part of a positive primary care relationship. DRL, on the other hand, coming from his training in analytic neutrality, wondered about the value of not accepting a gift, but instead examining the motive behind the gesture. This issue came up several times over the 9 years that DRL facilitated the group. He recollects that there was somewhat of an enduring conflict with some members who felt that it was not conducive to general practice to refuse and seek to understand, or interpret, a gift.

A similar difference between DRL and some group members emerged around the cases that involved a physician attending a patient's funeral. These were generally very positive experiences of appreciation and closure for the physician, but DRL commented at times from his analytic stance that for an analyst to attend a funeral often led to complex and contentious interactions with patients' families (RHP also had this experience at a funeral).

In other instances, two examples from DRL's time with the group helped to develop two key principles for the Boston group:

1   clarifying the professional boundaries that the facilitator needs to protect in the group; and
2   how at times the psychoanalytic notion of a termination may be of help to primary care doctors in stuck situations.

Several of the members of the early Boston Balint group had attended Rogerian-style (based on the methods of Carl Rogers) weekend workshops and had become enamored of the experience of occasional deep, personal enquiry from one member to another. One member began to explore the personal story behind another member's case presentation. The facilitator was perhaps not as quick to "head this off at the pass" as he had wished. The vulnerable member soon left the group and with DRL's help, the group "discovered" experientially the enduring value of Balint's imprecation against in-depth personal inquiries (Balint, 1965; Balint & Balint, 1962). The basic premise of residing in one's identity as a doctor (or any relationship-based profession, teacher, therapist) was annealed for the Boston Group and DRL through that experience.

The second example occurred on an occasion where a case involved a patient who just would not follow through on the doctor's advice and kept complaining of not getting better. DRL apparently (RHP only heard about this later when he was facilitating the group) offered the possible comment, "sometimes you might just have to say, 'that's all I can do for you.'" This apparently led to a positive outcome for the doctor and became a kind of group principle for "stuck" cases and had assumed the status of a basic tenet in the life of the Boston Group.

In my mind (RHP) as I think back to my years facilitating the Boston group, I often picture DRL facilitating the group in this early bridge area when he had been trained by Grete Bibring at Boston's Beth Israel, developing his life-long interest in the role psychiatry and psychoanalysis can play in medical care. He founded an Integration Clinic at Beth Israel, where psychiatrists, generalists, nurse practitioners and social workers all shared the same floor, so that collaborative care was occurring in the halls as well as in the offices (Lipsitt, 1964). RHP later inherited this clinic as it evolved, fueled by the support of the Federal government's primary care initiative, and importantly the Beth Israel's president, Doctor Mitchell Rabkin and the Chair of General Medicine, Doctor Tom Delbanco. It had expanded to become the ambulatory training site for all general internists and primary care residents, had 4 teams; each team had a team meeting, attended and facilitated by RHP, which often would turn into a Balint-like case discussion (with RHP's subtle introduction of Balint principles aiding in the containment of these case-based talks).

In about 1986 DRL and the group offered RHP the opportunity to take on the facilitator's role for the Boston Balint group. RHP graduated from BPSI in 1987 and his training had occurred during the advent of object relations, greater inclusion of ideas of Winnicott, Klein and Ferenczi. The adherence to anonymity and strict neutrality had evolved into an emphasis on the applied self psychology of Kohut and others. The transference was seen as the context for discussion; role responsiveness was emphasized. In short, psychoanalysis itself was moving away from instinct-based, interpretative certainty, more toward a developmental way of working that certainly included an unequivocal notion of the unconscious, but with less emphasis on deep genetic interpretation and more toward interactive, present moment, relationship-based observation of past patterns brought forward into the analytic space. This was very akin to the notions that Balint and Ferenczi had championed in Budapest in the 1920s and 1930s. It also was a return to an early technique paper of Freud's paper "Remembering, repeating and working through" (Freud, 1914).

Impact of Balint Groups on Participants, Patients and Leader

Current vitality of Balint Groups is validated by the increasing number of requests from practicing physicians as well as veterinarians and others. Of value to the community involvement of modern psychoanalysts is the way in which Balint leadership training has been nurtured for the last 30 years largely by the International Balint Federation (IBF) and the American Balint Society (ABS). For the present-day psychoanalyst, trained for the most part in object relations, relational theory and field theory, there exists a recognizable dynamic in the structure and process of a present-day Balint group (Balint & Balint, 1955).

The absence of genetic interpretations, of deep interpretations in general, the avoidance of interpretive authority, the primacy of empathy, reverie, shared discovery of meaning, containment of conflict, are predominant in the Balint group, as well as in a psychoanalysis conducted in 2020. By 1966, with a decade of experience in running groups for British primary care physicians and publishing Psychoanalysis and medical practice, Balint had contributed profoundly to healing this rift by bringing an integrative method that used psychoanalytic principles in ways that did not offend but rather invited physicians' personal experiences to a learning process group (Balint, 1954).

The Future of Balint Groups

Emergence of New Applications of Psychoanalysis to Medicine

The 1930s and early 1940s saw the emergence of a group of medical psychoanalysts with a growing interest in psychosomatic medicine. They began writing of the ways in which psychoanalytic concepts might help general physicians improve their comprehension of their relationships to patients. Flanders Dunbar (1935), credited with the origins of the American Psychosomatic Society (1942) and the journal *Psychosomatic Medicine* (1939), Carl Binger (1945) and Franz Alexander (1950), who had been a pupil of Ferenczi, were early investigators. Bertram Lewin in 1946 wrote "recent medical literature has introduced many psychoanalytic concepts to the larger medical world, among others that of the transference" (Lewin, 1946, p. 195). Other psychoanalysts who took great interest in the growing popularity of psychosomatic medicine included Felix and Helene Deutsch, Leon Salzburg, Edward and Grete Bibring, as well as several other psychoanalyst emigres from war-threatened Europe. Most of the articles published in early issues of *Psychosomatic Medicine* were by psychoanalysts applying new ideas to an understanding of physical illness.

The question persists whether Balint Groups will be able to continue in the format originally established by Michael Balint (Ornstein, 2002). He had begun his work when circumstances were propitious for success. In 1924, he had been recruited in Hungary by general practitioners eager to improve their experience (and perhaps their esteem) treating patients and enjoying the patina of association with a psychoanalyst at a time that might enhance their own image. In Britain in the 1950s, conditions were different. Psychosomatic medicine had made an impression on the public as a way of integrating concepts of both body and mind and had generated considerable interest in physicians who had recently returned from a war experience where they had witnessed firsthand the benefits of a holistic approach to treatment. GPs tended to be regarded as lower on the medical totem pole. Balint exuded a special affiliation with practicing physicians; he was a man of generous, creative and friendly character (Lipsitt, 1999). He did not use psychoanalytic jargon, but chose innovative ways of speaking of "the drug doctor," "investment in the physician- patient relationship," and the patient's background and family as his or her "account." The concept has continued to appeal to some physicians over the years, either those who already possessed receptive attitudes about the psychological aspects of patient care, or those who sought the camaraderie of other like-minded physicians with whom they could share the stresses and strains of quotidian practice. Research into doctor–patient relationships begun by Michael and Enid Balint continues to advance (Tschuschke & Flatten, 2019).

Contemporary medicine has whittled away much "leisure" time of the physician, increasingly imposing greater responsibility, resulting, some say, in wide prevalence of "burnout" and dissatisfactions with the health care system. The need for support and comfort persists, perhaps with a pandemic and other challenges, but may now appear in modified forms and "names." Institutions like Kaiser-Permanente have promoted volunteer gatherings in groups called "Connect the Docs," or "Meaning in Medicine" (E. D. Lipsitt, personal communication) where physicians can discuss cases, let off steam, or simply enjoy the company and support of professional colleagues. What started out with psychoanalyst facilitator/leaders has been supplanted over the years with general practitioners, family doctors, psychiatrists and other professionals with interests in the value of group interaction. In the Dutch experience, general practitioners were reported to have difficulty finding anyone who would accept the responsibility of leader (Main, 1979, p. 268). Nevertheless, Michael Balint's legacy remains an instructive model in extolling the value of group interaction for teaching, learning, growth and pleasure.

Balint's seminal contributions are not limited to his work with general physicians. The story of consultation-liaison (C-L) psychiatry owes a debt to Michael Balint for paving the way toward a dedicated psychodynamic two-person approach to understanding the patient–doctor relationship (Lipsitt, 2017). He pioneered a way of translating psychoanalytic percepts into language that could be understood, enjoyed and applied to C-L work (Kahana & Bibring, 1956). He also helped to devise an approach to "focal" psychotherapy, an essential aspect of interviewing medical/surgical patients with whom the psychiatrist must sometimes make psychodynamic assessments in the briefest of interactions (Blacher, 1984). Towards the end of Balint's life, in collaboration with Winnicott, he was elaborating a concept of rapid, informed technique called the "flash" for physicians who did not have the luxury of "the long interview." Further described posthumously in the book, *Six Minutes for the Patient* (Balint & Norell, 1973), this innovative scheme has become invaluable to the practicing consulting psychiatrist who must often make useful recommendations with limited time and data. A prescient example of such an approach is exquisitely illustrated in Freud's case of Katharina (Freud, 1895; Breuer & Freud, 1895, pp. 125–134; Lipsitt, 2017, pp. 86–87).

Recitative

The quest for a more humanistic approach to medicine has existed for decades, especially as "scientific" and biological medicine reach further and further into the genomic, physiological and anatomical bases of medical practice. Psychiatry and psychoanalysis may be said to have evolved in part from a wish to preserve the individual as more than a mere assemblage of body parts, electric and neurocirculatory systems. It was Michael Balint's desire to help physicians in interaction with their patients to retain a holistic understanding of their relationships (Paulsen, 2019). In his usual direct and unencumbered way, Balint is quoted in front matter of Hopkins's book: "It happens so rarely in life that you have a person who understands what you are up to and openly faces it with you. That is what we can do for our patients and it is an enormous thing" (Hopkins, 1979).

The basic premise of all therapies is to help individuals integrate mind and body to optimal efficiency allowing for satisfactory adaptation to one's own satisfaction, relative happiness and social demands. Physicians, through participation in Balint groups, have been aided in accepting this responsibility and commitment to do no harm. That primary care physicians should or can become junior psychiatrists capable of providing psychotherapy within the confines of their daily practice has long been debated. There is neither time, skill nor inclination for this to happen. As emphasized by Burke, White and Havens (1979), "when a patient's resources of time, money, or motivation are limited, psychotherapists face the problem of how to be effective in a brief period of time" (p. 177). Unfortunately, there is much about health care that simply cannot be hurried. Balint's approach intended to make "second-messengers" of practicing physicians who could alter the way general medicine is practiced. It has not been denied that physicians can, if so inclined, learn how to use the usual time per patient for a more empathic, sensitive, deeper understanding of a patient's whole illness experience to considerable benefit for the patient and even the likelihood of more satisfaction for the physician.

What might almost be an epitaph for Michael Balint, an appreciation of Michael Balint (Lakising, 2005, p. 724) noted simply "One of the most notable names in general practice, Michael Balint's analysis of the doctor–patient relationship and use of group therapy made him an internationally acclaimed figure." More expansively, Balint was also described "At once a doctor, psychotherapist, teacher, writer and humanist, Michael Balint surely ranks among the most influential medical figures of the 20th century." Of note, both encomiums omit the title psychoanalyst (ibid., p. 725). Doctor Tom Main perhaps captured the overarching theme of Balint's work: "If we all listen to each other, we have to hear from each other" (Hopkins, 1979, p. 270).

Note

The interested reader can learn more about the American Balint Society (ABS), its mission, structure, leadership training programs and certification process, free short-term online Balint groups and annual meetings at its website (https://americanbalintsociety.org). The ABS provides current assurance that the basic discoveries and tenets of Balint work continue in the future.

References

Alexander, F. (1950). *Psychosomatic medicine.* New York: W.W. Norton & Co.
Alexander, F. & French, T.M. (1946). *Psychoanalytic therapy: principles and applications.* New York: Ronald Press.
Anzieu, D. (2001). Freud's group psychology. In E.S. Person (Ed.), *On Freud's "Group psychology and the analysis of the ego"* (pp. 39–60). Hillside, NJ: The Analytic Press.
Balint, E. & Norell, J.S. (1973). *Six minutes for the patient.* London: Tavistock Publications.
Balint, M. (1923). On the psychotherapies for the practicing physician. *Therapie,* 5.
Balint, M. (1926). Psychoanalysis and clinical medicine. *Zeitschrift fur Klinische Medizen,* 103, 628.
Balint, M. (1933a). (Obituary). Sandor Ferenczi. *International Journal of Psychoanalysis,* 30, 215–219.
Balint, M. (1933b). Dr. Sandor Ferenczi as psychoanalyst. In M. Balint (Ed.), *Problems of human pleasure and behavior* (pp. 235–242). New York: Liveright.
Balint, M. (1948). Sandor Ferenczi. In M. Balint (Ed.), *Problems of human pleasure and behavior* (pp. 243–250). New York: Liveright.
Balint, M. (1954). Training general practitioners in psychotherapy. *British Medical Journal,* 1, 115–120.
Balint, M. (1956). Individual differences in behavior and early infancy and an objective method of recording them. In M. Balint, *Problems of human pleasure and behavior.* New York: Liveright.
Balint, M. (1957a). *The doctor, his patient and the illness.* London: Pitman Medical.
Balint, M. (1957b). Psychotherapy and the general practitioner. *British Medical Journal,* 1, 156–158.
Balint, M. (1958). Sandor Ferenczi's last years. *International Journal of Psychoanalysis,* 39, 68.
Balint, M. (1960). The marital problem clinic – a problem child of the F.P.A. *Family Planning,* 9, 18–20.
Balint, M. (1961a). The other part of medicine. *Lancet,* 1, 40–42.
Balint, M. (1961b). *Psychotherapeutic techniques in medicine.* London: Tavistock Publications.
Balint, M. (1968). *The basic fault: Therapeutic aspects of regression.* London: Tavistock Publications.
Balint, M. (1965). The doctor's therapeutic function. *Lancet,* 1, 1177–1180.
Balint, M. (1966). Psycho-analysis and medical practice. *International Journal of Psychoanalysis,* 47, 54–62.
Balint, M. (1970). Repeat prescription patients: are they an identifiable group? *International Journal of Psychiatry in Medicine,* 1, 3–14.

Balint, M. (2002). The crisis of medical practice. *American Journal of Psychoanalysis*, 62(1), 7–15.
Balint, M. & Balint, E. (1955). Dynamics of training in groups for psychotherapy. *British Journal of Medical Psychology*, 28, 135–142.
Balint, M. & Balint, E. (1962). *Psychotherapeutic techniques in medicine*. London: Tavistock/Lippincott.
Balint, M., Balint, E., Gosling, R. & Hildebrand, P. (1966). *A study of doctors*. London: Tavistock Publications.
Balint, M., Ornstein, P.H. & Balint, E. (1972). *Focal psychotherapy: An example of applied psychoanalysis*. London: Tavistock/Lippincott.
Bibring, G.L. (1956). Psychiatry and medical practice in a general hospital. *New England Journal of Medicine*, 254(8), 366–372.
Binger, C. (1945). *The doctor's job*. New York: W.W. Norton & Co.
Bion, W.R. (1961). *Experiences in groups*. London: Tavistock Publications.
Blacher, R. (1984). The briefest encounter: psychotherapy for medical and surgical patients. *General Hospital Psychiatry*, 6(3), 226–232.
Breuer, J. & Freud, S. (1895). *Studies on hysteria*. New York: Basic Books.
Burke, J.D., White, H.S. & Havens, L.L. (1979). Which short term therapy? *Archives of General Psychiatry*, 36(2), 177–186.
Dimitrijevic, A., Casullo, G. & Frankel, J. (2018). *Ferenczi's influence on contemporary psychoanalytic traditions: Lines of development, evolution of theory and practice over the decades*. New York: Routledge.
Dunbar, F. (1935). *Emotions and bodily changes*. New York: Columbia University Press.
Engel, L. (2020). Michael Balint, his life and work. Retrieved from balintsrbija.org. Accessed July 23.
Family Discussion Bureau. (1955). *Social casework in marital problems: The development of a psychodynamic approach*. London: Tavistock Publications.
Ferenczi, S. (1980a [1921]). *First contributions to psychoanalysis*. New York: Brunner/Mazel.
Ferenczi, S. (1980b). *Further contributions to the theory and the techniques of psychoanalysis*. New York: Brunner/Mazel.
Ferenczi, S. (1982). Presentation abregee de la psychoanalyse. *Psychoanalyse*, 4, 148–194.
Ferenczi, S. (1984a). *Final contributions to the problems and methods of psychoanalysis*. London: Karnac Books.
Ferenczi, S. (1984b). Freud's influence on medicine. In S. Ferenczi, *Final contributions to the problems and methods of psychoanalysis*. (pp. 143–155). London: Karnac Books.
Ferenczi, S. (1923). La psychoanaklyse au service de l'omnopraction. Presentation at Kassa.
Ferenczi, S. & Rank, O. (1923). *The development of psycho-analysis*. New York: Nervous and Mental Disease Publishing Company.
Freud, S. (1895). Katharina. In J. Breuer & S. Freud, *Studies on hysteria* (pp. 125–134). New York: Basic Books. 1957.
Freud, S. (1904). On psychotherapy. In J. Strachey (Ed.) [1953], *The standard edition of the complete psychological works of Sigmund Freud*, volume 7 (pp. 255–268). London: Hogarth Press.

Freud, S. (1913) Totem and Taboo and other works. In J. Strachey (Ed.) [1955], *The standard edition of the complete psychological works of Sigmund Freud*, volume 13 (pp. 1–255). London: Hogarth Press.

Freud, S. (1914). Remembering, repeating and working through. In J. Strachey (Ed.) [1958], *The standard edition of the complete psychological works of Sigmund Freud*, volume 12 (pp. 147–156). London: Hogarth Press.

Freud, S. (1919). Lines of advance in psychoanalytic therapy. In J. Strachey (Ed.) [1955], *The standard edition of the complete psychological works of Sigmund Freud*, volume 17 (pp. 157–168). London: Hogarth Press.

Freud, S. (1924). Sandor Ferenczi. *International Journal of Psychoanalysis*, 14, 207.

Freud, S. (1925, 1926). The question of lay analysis and other works. An autobiographical study, inhibition, symptoms and anxiety. In J. Strachey (Ed.) [1954], *The standard edition of the complete psychological works of Sigmund Freud*, volume 20 (pp. 1–192). London: Hogarth Press.

Gendrot, J-A. (1972). In memoriam. In P. Hopkins (Ed.) *Patient-centred medicine* (pp. 300–304). London: Regional Doctor Publications.

Gosling, R. (1966). History. In M. Balint, E. Balint, R. Gosling & P. Hildebrand (Eds.), *A study of doctors*. London: Tavistock/Lippincott.

Hopkins, P. (1972). Interview of Michael Balint (November 27, 1970). In P. Hopkins, *Patient-centred medicine* (pp. 316–326). London: Regional Doctor Publications.

Hopkins, P. (1979). *The human face of medicine*. London: Pitman Medical.

Kahana, R.J. & Bibring, G.L. (1956). Personality types in medical management. In N. E. Zinberg (Ed.). *Psychiatry and medical practice in a general hospital* (pp. 108–123). New York: International Universities Press.

Knoepfel, H-K. (1972). The effects of the Balint group on its members and leader. *International Journal of Psychiatry in Medicine*, 3, 379–383.

Lacan, J. (2001). The function and field of speech and language in psychoanalysis. In J. Lacan (Ed.), *A selection* (pp. 33–125). London: Routledge.

Lakising, E. (2005) Michael Balint, an outstanding medical life: An appreciation of Michael Balint. *British Journal of General Practice*, 55(518), 724–725.

Levine, M. (1957). Forward. In M. Balint, *The doctor, his patient and the illness*. New York: International Universities Press.

Lewin, B. (1946). Counter-transference in the technique of medical practice. *Psychosomatic Medicine*, 8, 195–199.

Lipsitt, D.R. (2020). In Freud's pocket: A totem of Freud's ambivalence toward medicine? *American Imago*, 77(4), 738–751.

Lipsitt, D.R. (2017). *Foundations of consultation-liaison psychiatry: the bumpy road to specialization*. New York: Routledge.

Lipsitt, D.R. (1999). Michael Balint's group approach: The Boston Balint group. *Group*, 23, 187–201.

Lipsitt, D.R. (1964). Integration Clinic: An approach to the teaching and practice of medical psychology in an outpatient setting. In N.E. Zinberg (Ed.), *Psychiatry and medical practice in a general hospital* (pp. 231–249). New York: International Universities Press.

Main, T. (1979). Epilogue. In P. Hopkins (Ed.), *The human face of medicine* (pp. 265–270) Kent: Pitman Publishing.

Malan, D.H. (1963). *A study of brief psychotherapy*. London: Tavistock/Lippincott.

Moreau-Ricaud, M. (2015). Filiation Freud-Ferenczi-Balint: faith and evolution in psychoanalysis. *Connexions*, 2(104), 149–164.

Norquist, G.S. & Regier, D.A. (1996). The epidemiology of psychiatric disorders and the de facto mental health care system. *Annual Review of Medicine*, 47, 473–479.

Oppenheim-Gluckman, H. (2015). *Reading Michael Balint: a pragmatic clinician*. New York: Routledge.

Ornstein, P.H. (2002). Michael Balint then and now: a contemporary appraisal. *American Journal of Psychoanalysis*, 62(1), 25–35.

Paulsen, R.H. (1996). Psychiatry and primary care as neighbors; from the Promethean primary care physician to multidisciplinary clinic. *International Journal of Psychiatry in Medicine*, 26(2), 113–125.

Paulsen, R.H. (1997). What would primary care providers like from us? *Psychotherapy Forum*, 4(2).

Paulsen, R.H. (2019). Balint, psychoanalysis and primary care medicine. Podcast, June 9. Retrieved from ipaoffthecouch.org (accessed November 21, 2020).

Player, M., Freedy, J.R., Diaz, V. et al. (2018). The role of Balint group training in the professional development of family medicine residents. *International Journal of Psychiatry in Medicine*, 53, 24–38.

Rachman, A.W. (1999). Ferenczi's rise and fall from "analytic grace": The Ferenczi renaissance revisited. *Group*, 23(3/4), 103–119.

Raimbault, G. (1979). Aims of training and medical ideals. In P. Hopkins (Ed.), *The human face of medicine* (pp. 26–28). Kent: Pitman Publishing.

Schacht, L. (1977). Introduction. In G. Groddeck, *The meaning of illness: selected psychoanalytic writings* (pp. 1–28). London: Hogarth Press.

Smith, R.C. (2011). Educating trainees about common mental health problems in primary care: a (not so) modest proposal. *Academic Medicine*, 86(11), e16.

Smith, R.C., Laird-Fick, H., D'Mello, D., Dwamena, F.C.et al. (2014). Addressing mental health issues in primary care: an initial curriculum for medical residents. *Patient Education and Counseling*, 94(1), 33–42.

Stewart, H. (1989). Technique of the basic fault/regression. *International Journal of Psychoanalysis*, 70, 221–230.

Stewart, H. et al. (1996). *Michael Balint, object relations pure and applied*. London: Routledge.

Swerdloff, B. (2002). An interview with Michael Balint. *American Journal of Psychoanalysis*, 62(4), 383–413.

Tschuschke, V. & Flatten, G. (2019). Effect of group leaders on doctors' learning in Balint groups. *International Journal of Psychiatry in Medicine*, 54, 83–96.

Wikipedia. (2021). Ronald Fairbairn. Retrieved from https://en.wikipedia.org/wiki/Ronald_Fairbairn.

Winnicott, D.W. (1963). The development of the capacity for concern. In D.W. Winnicott, *The maturational process and the facilitating environment* (pp. 73–78). London: Routledge.

Winnicott, D.W. (1966). Psycho-somatic illness in its positive and negative aspects. *International Journal of Psychoanalysis*, 47, 510–516.

Winnicott, D. W. (1984). The observation of infants in a setting situation. In D.W. Winnicott (Ed.), *Through paediatrics to psychoanalysis* (pp. 52–69). London: Karnac Books.

Index

A-Team, The (TV series) 58, 59
abandonment anxiety/trauma 16, 74, 86, 138, 148
ABS (American Balint Society) 172, 175, 182, 185–186
acting-out behaviors 73, 74, 75, 76, 80, 81, 86
Adams Silvan, Abby 104
addiction 4–5, 129–135; and dehumanization 5, 126, 133, 134–135, 139; and dependence/independence 125–127, 133, 139; literature gap for 137; and mental representations 133–134; and object relations 125, 132–133, 134, 138; and therapeutic distance 137–138; and therapeutic relationship 5, 129, 130–132, 135–138; and transference/countertransference 128, 134, 135–136, 138, *see also* alcohol abuse; substance abuse
adolescence 4, 80–81, 91–92, 94, 96
affect equivalents 9
affect regulation 3, 72, 77, 80, 117, 134
Albanese, M.J. 133
alcohol abuse 13, 15
Alexander, Franz 172, 173–174, 183
alexithymia 9–10, 80, 149
allergies 5, 142, 143, 148–149
alpha function 117–118, 119
American Balint Society (ABS) 172, 175, 182, 185–186
anger 55, 57, 94, 98, 99, 120, 135, 136, 143
anorexia nervosa 8, 12–14, 21, 74, 75–76, 82, 87, 91–93; and dynamic psychiatry 93–94; and families 92–93, 94, 99; medication for 94; and pain 97, 98, 99; pediatric aspects of 95; and suicide risk 93–94; symptoms/diagnosis of 91–92, 95
anxieties 103, 119, 179; abandonment 74; of clinician 27, 28, 33, 34, 35; of parents 28–29
Anzieu, D. 147, 149
Arcimboldo, Giuseppe 145
Aristotle 22
Athens Maternity Hospital project 44–49; aim of 45; impact of 45–47; parents' testimonies 48–49; theoretical references of 44–45
attachment 79–80, 82, 118–120
attachment theory 77, 126
autonomy 66, 67, 126

Balint, Alice (née Szekely-Kovacs) 164, 165, 170
Balint, Enid (née Eichholz) 52, 66, 165, 171, 175, 184
Balint, Michael 5, 161–174, 179, 180, 183; career 165–167; early life 163–165; father 163–164, 165, 168, 169, 174; and Ferenczi 161, 164, 165, 166–171; and focal/applied psychotherapy 174, 184; and GPs 161, 162, 163, 164, 166, 168, 169–171, 172; legacy of 184–185; as outsider 169; and third watershed *see* third watershed
Balint Groups 5, 27, 167, 171–172, 173, 174–185; components of 176; and feelings of physicians 176–177, 178, 179; future of 183–185; impact of 182–183; and information exchange 180; and patients' funerals 177, 178, 181; procedure of 175–177; and professional boundaries 179, 181; and relational/field theories 175; role of

presenter in 175, 177;
supporting/holding role of 178–179;
and termination in stuck situations
181; in US 180–182, 185–186
Becker, Ernst 105–106
Beranger, Madeleine/Beranger, Willy 128
bereavement 111, 112, 113, 116, 120, 178–179
Bergman, T. 51
Berlin (Germany) 164, 165–166
beta elements 117, 118, 119
Beth Israel Hospital, Boston (US) 181–182
Bibring, Grete 174, 181, 183
Bick, Esther 24
binge eating 94, 130, 131, 132, 138
Binger, Carl 183
Bion, Wilfred 25, 30, 117–118, 119, 171, 172, 173
blame 2, 30, 59, 131
Blatt, Sydney 79
Bluebond-Langner, M. 57
board game 63–65, *64*, 66, 69
body image 3, 6, 8, 73, 74, 76–80, 81, 94, 159; and cultural influence 78; and depression 79; and early development 77; and failed mirroring 77–79; and insecure attachment 79–80; and physical/sexual abuse 79; and sense of self 76–77, 78–79, 80, 82
body scheme 156, 159
Bollas, C. 68
bone marrow transplants 59, 60, 61, 65, 66, 68, 69
borderline disorders 10, 73, 77, 87
Boston Balint Group 180–182
Bower, M. 133, 137
Bowlby, John 24, 119, 125–126, 172–173
Boyd, William 51, 66
BPO (borderline personality organizations) 73, 87
Breitbart, William 106
Brenner, Charles 133
Breuer, J. 9, 163
Britain (UK) 52, 72, 101, 104, 164–165, 166, 170, 171–172
British Independents 172–174
British Psychoanalytic Society 24, 170, 172
Budapest (Hungary) 164, 166–167, 168, 170, 182

Buenos Aires (Argentina) 1, 72, 157;
Children's General Hospital Ricardo Gutiérrez 4, 91, 95–97
bulimia 73, 74, 76, 82, 87, 94, 95
Burke, J.D. 185
Bydlowski, M. 42

C-L (consultation-liaison) psychiatry 184
Caillois, Roger 156
cancer 4, 55–69, 113–116, 178; and therapeutic relationship 56–61, 62, 63, 65–66, *see also* psycho-oncology
Castelnuovo-Tedesco, P. 60–61
cathexis 11, 121
CBT (cognitive-behavioral therapies) 80
Centro Studi Martha Harris (Florence) 2, 24
chemotherapy 61, 107, 114, 115, 118
child guidance clinics 24, 166, 170, 172
children 3, 24, 26, 172; and depression 40; drawings by 63–65, *64*, 113; and eating disorders *see* eating disorders; history of mental health care for 95–96; and pain 2; terminally ill 61–66, 113, *see also* pediatric wards
Children's General Hospital Ricardo Gutiérrez (Buenos Aires) 4, 91, 95–99; eating disorder patient case study 97–99; history of Mental Health Unit 95–96; therapeutic model of 96–97
chronic illness 15, 16–18, 19, 22
co-creation 43–44, 46
cognitive-behavioral therapies (CBT) 80
Cohen, Margaret 53, 67
communities 1, 84–85, 106, 113
compassion 4, 102, 114, 115, 135
complementarity 127–128
conflict theory 77
Connor, Steven 146, 150, 153
constellative psychomatics 8
consultation-liaison (C-L) psychiatry 184
containment 25, 29, 33, 96, 182
conversion psychosomatic model 8–9
coping mechanisms 59, 67, 115
countertransference 5, 16, 25, 73, 75–76, 103, 105, 169, 174; and addiction 128, 134, 138; and palliative care 111, 114
Courage to Survive, The (film) 104
COVID-19 15
Crohn's Disease 18–21; adaptations to 19–20

Davids, J. 51
day hospital (DH) programs 71–87; and abandonment anxiety 74; and body image 77, 80–81; and borderline patients 73; and bulimic patients 73, 74, 76, 82, 87; commensality in 85; and communities 71, 77, 84, 85; contract-based approach in 73; and embodiment experiences 81, 87; and global treatment strategy 85, 87; goals/framework 83–85; group approach in 73, 74, 75, 77, 85; and individualism 84; interdisciplinary approach in 71, 72, 83, 84; management of cases in 72–73; mentalization-based treatment in 74, 77, 81–83, 87; and milieu therapy 72, 85; as out of the couch therapy 81, 83, 84; psychodynamic approach in 71, 72, 73, 77, 80, 84–85, 86–87; and representation of emotions 76; supervision in 73, 75, 76; and therapeutic community 72, 75, 84, 85; and transference/countertransference 75–76, 83, 85
dead mother 127, 134
death 111, 153, *see also* palliative care
death anxiety 4, 16, 20, 101, 104–109, 112, 119; case study 107–109; literature on 105–106; and value/meaning 106–107, *see also* existential maturity
death drive 119, 121
decathexis 121, 128
deep brain stimulation 6
defense mechanism theory 77
defenses 30, 68, 79, 114, 115
dehumanization 5, 102, 126, 133, 134–135, 139; and dead mother 127
denial 4, 19, 20, 29, 105, 108, 109, 133
dependence 5, 15, 125–127, 133, 139
depression 15, 19, 56, 74, 75, 79, 103, 135; in children 40; and eating disorders 75, 76, 79, 81, 93; and pregnant women 36–37
depressive position 118, 120
dermatitis 143, 148, 149, 150, 156
dermatologists 5, 141, 146, 147–148, 153, 154, 157
Desmarais, J. 68
Deutsch, Felix 166, 168, 183
DH programs *see* day hospital programs

diagnosis 12, 14
dichotomous thinking 2, 10, 22, 141, 145
directed phenomena 156
disseminative encephalomyelitis 7–8
distress 26–27; functional/behavioral 31–32
drugs *see* addiction
Dunbar, Flanders 183
dynamic thinking 2
dysphoria 74, 134, 138

eating disorders (ED) 3–4, 71–87, 91–99; and acting-out behaviors 73, 74, 75, 76, 80, 81; anorexia *see* anorexia nervosa; and attachment theory 77, 79–80, 82; binge eating 94, 130, 131, 132; and body image *see* body image; bulimia 73, 74, 76, 82, 87, 94, 95; and depressive symptoms 75, 76, 79, 81; DH programs for *see* day hospital (DH) programs; and emptiness/withdrawal 74, 79; and families 92–93, 94, 97, 99; and feeling/thinking problem 75, 76, 80, 81; and girls/femininity 80–81; hospital program for *see* Children's General Hospital Ricardo Gutiérrez; and interdisciplinary approach 71, 72, 83, 84, 91, 93, 99; literature on 71; medication for 94; pediatric aspects of 95; persistent enduring (EED) 72, 74, 75, 79, 81, 83; and primitive states/defenses 75, 77, 80, 86–87; and sexual abuse 74, 79, 80–81; and suicide risk 74, 80, 81, 93–94; symptoms/diagnosis of 91–92, 95
eczema 142, 144, 152
ego 11, 142, 149, 150, 151, 152, 155, 176; regression 19; restrictions 10; and somatic illness 16, 19
Eichholz, Enid (later Balint) 52, 66, 165, 171, 175
embodiment experiences 81, 87
Emmanuel, R. 59
emotional immersion 2, 25
empathy 4, 61, 67, 102, 109, 152, 158, 182, 185
emptiness 74, 79, 130, 138; and terminally ill patients 115, 116, 121
encephalomyelitis 7–8, 16–17
Engel, George 6–7
Erikson, E.H. 113

eroticism/erotic body 78, 80, 141, 142, 155, 157
Escardó, Florencio 96
euphoria 7–8
existential maturity 112–113, 118, 119, 120–121, 122; and age 113; and groups/intersubjectivity 113; of therapists 123
existential psychoanalysis 105–106

Fairburn, W.R.D. 126, 133, 138, 172
families 2, 4, 20–21, 68–69, 106–107, 171; and eating disorders 92–93, 94, 97, 99; and palliative care 113, 113–114, 119, 121; and skin patients 144, 148, 154–155
family therapy 75, 96, 97, 98–99
fathers 3, 13, 29, 43, 48, 129, 168; absent 97, 99; and jealousy 31, 33
feminine 80–81, 93
Fenichel, Otto 9
Ferenczi, Sandor 5, 161, 164, 165, 166–171, 174, 182, 183
field theory 175, 182
"flash" technique 184
Florence (Italy) 2, 24, 26
Flores, Philip 125
fluoxetine 94, 108
focal psychotherapy 174, 184
Fonagy, Peter 77, 81–82
fragmentation 121
Frankl, Viktor 106
free association 5, 163, 169, 171, 176, 177
French Balint Society 163, 172
Freud, Anna 51
Freud, Sigmund 25, 96, 125, 158, 182; and Balint Groups 5, 164, 166, 168, 169, 182, 184; and complementarity 127–128; and death/mourning 105, 121, 147; and psychosomatic approach 8–9, 141–142, 143, 146, 148, 162–163, 168, 169–170, 173, 175
funerals, patients' 177, 178, 181
Furman, E. 65

gastric banding 6
gastric ulcers 6
Gauchet, Marcel 83–84
gaze, the 5, 55–58, 142, 143
Gendrot, J-A. 163
general practitioners *see* GPs

Gieler, U. 149
gift-giving, patients' 65, 66, 180–181
Gill, Richard 125
Goldie, L. 68
GPs (general practitioners) 161, 162, 163–164, 166, 168, 169–171, 172; and modern health care system 184, *see also* Balint Groups
grandparents 21, 30, 56, 68, 114, 115, 117, 148, 149
Greece 36, 38, 44, *see also* Athens Maternity Hospital project
Green, Andre 79, 121, 127, 134, 145, 151, 155
grief 101, 102, 103, 104, 112, 121, 122
Groddeck, Georg 168–169
group therapy 73, 74, 75, 77, 85, 96, 97, 98, 173, *see also* Balint Groups
guilt 30, 34, 54, 67

Harris, Martha 24, 25
Havens, L.L. 185
Heidelberg Research Project *see* Crohn's Disease
Helicobacter 6
helplessness: of medical staff 54, 61; of patients 68; of therapist 30, 34, 53, 55, 62, 66
hero myth 175
historization 86, 91
holding environment 115, 127, 168, 172, 179
holistic approach 46, 47, 183, 185
Holland, Jimmie 101
homeostasis 6, 141
Hopkins, P. 163, 164, 185
Houlding, S. 66
Hungary 163–164, 165, 166, 173, 182, 183
hypochondria 10, 11, 12, 103
hysteria 8, 9, 141, 162, 163

Iacoboni, Marco 12
IBF (International Balint Federation) 182
identity 60, 61, 81, 127–128; and skin patients 142, 149, 150, 153, 156
identity diffusion 21, 73, 77, 87
immigrants 38
impulsivity 73, 74, 75, 81
independence 125, 126, 133, 139
indexical function of body 9

individualism 84
infant abuse 37–38
infant mortality 38
infant observation 24, 25, 49
infants 2, 3; and depressive position 118, 120; and object relations 127, 133–134; premature *see* premature infants
infant–mother relationship 3, 25, 118, 171, 175; and attachment process 77, 79–80, 82, 126; and depression 37; and holding 127; and mentalization 77; and mirror neurons 152; and mirroring 78; in pregnancy 41–42; and premature infants 39, 40–41; and therapeutic relationship 168
interdisciplinary approach 71, 72, 83, 84, 91, 93, 96, 99, 146, 147–148
International Balint Federation (IBF) 182
interventional methods 6, 41–48
introspection 76
IPA (International Psychoanalytic Association) 1
Italy 2, 24, 26

jealousy 21, 31, 33
Jeammet, Philippe 74, 82
Jeannet, P. 92
Johnson, Brian 133

Katz, D.A. 56, 67
Kernberg, Otto 73
Kernberg, Paulina 78
Kestemberg, J. 92–93
Khantzian, E.J. 133, 137, 138
Klein, Melanie 25, 118, 119, 133, 170, 182
Knoepfel, H-K. 161
Kohut, Heinz 126, 182

Lacan, J. 157–158
learning 24–26; from experience 24–25
leukaemia 56–66, 67–69
Leuzinger-Bohleber, Marianne 77
Lévi-Strauss, Claude 144, 147
Levine, M. 172
Lewin, Bertram 183
Liberman, David 155
Lipsitt, Don 180–182
listening, insightful/immersive 1–2, 67

Loewald, H.W. 128
loneliness 74, 79
love 111, 120, 148
Ludwig, M.W.B. 156

McDougall, Joyce 133, 148, 154
Magin, P. 157
Manchester (UK) 164–165, 170
manic state/episodes 15–16
masochism 143, 148, 156
maturity *see* existential maturity
MBT (mentalization-based treatment) 74, 77, 81–83, 87
meaning-making 116–121, 122, 145; and attachment styles 118–120; and Bion/Klein 117–118; limitations of 121; and oscillating positions/transitional space 118, 120–121
medical practitioners *see* MPs
Meltzer, Donald 24
mentalization 3, 74, 77, 81–83, 87; embodied 83
mentalization-based treatment (MBT) 74, 77, 81–83, 87
Metzger, Eran 180
midwives 46–47
mimetic moment 151
mind/body *see* somato-psychic dimension
Minuchin, S. 93
mirror neurons 151–152
mirroring 77–79, 81, 115
Moreau-Ricaud, M. 164
mothers 13, 14, 115–116, 129, 135; and anxiety 29; of eating disorder patients 92–93, 97, 99
mothers, new 36, 48–49; and body-to-body connection 3, 41, 42; and premature infants *see* premature infants; psychodynamic interventions for 41–48, *see also* perinatal depression; perinatal period
mourning *see* grief
MPs (medical practitioners) 11, 12, 22, *see also* GPs
multidisciplinary approach 43, 44, 45, 49–50, 71

narcissism 3, 77, 78, 92, 108, 167
Nazis 164, 165, 173
Nemiah, J.C. 10

neonatal intensive care units (NICUs) 37, 38–41, 42–43, 53
neuroscience 31, 42, 79
neurosis 9–10, 92
non-compliance 16–18
non-verbal communication 53, 68
Norton, J. 66

object constancy 134
object relations 2, 7, 10, 14, 17, 120, 121, 122, 127, 172, 182; and addiction 125, 132–133, 138
observation 18, 25, 26, 30, 35, 53, 173; clinical 49, 77, 87
omnipotence 4, 34, 46, 47, 74, 86, 134
On the Edge of Being (film) 102
oncologists 101–102
Oppenheim-Gluckmann, H. 166, 168, 170
Ornstein, Paul/Ornstein, Anna 171
oscillating positions 34–35, 118, 120–121
out of the couch therapy 81, 83, 84

pain 2, 33, 97, 98, 99, 129, 131, 138
palliative care 4, 111–123; and conceptions of death 112, 115–117, 121; distinctive features of 122; and existential maturity *see* existential maturity; and families 113, 113–114; and meaning-making 116–121; psychodynamic approach to 112, 114, 116, 122; and relationships 119, 120, 121, 122; and transference/countertransference 111, 114
panic attacks 19, 107, 108
paranoid schizoid position 120
Parens, H. 125
parents 13, 26–27, 28–31, 121, 129; of children with eating disorders 77–78, 93; new *see* perinatal period
patient-centred medicine 172
Paulsen, Randy 180
pediatric wards 51–69; cancer patient case studies 56–69; coping mechanisms in 59, 67; death of children in 66, 68, 69; distress of children in 57–59, 61, 62, 67, 68; emotions of staff in 54, 55–56, 61, 65, 66, 67; and families 53, 54, 56; and inner work of therapist 66–67; patient's board game in 63–65, *64*, 66,

69; and patients' search for meaning 68; regression in 52, 61, 66, 67–68; relations between staff in 53–54, 66; role of psychotherapy in 51–52, 53, 61, 66, 67–68
pediatricians/pediatrics 2, 24, 26–35, 49, 96, 98; and anxiety 27, 28, 33, 34, 35; and containment 29, 33; and fatigue/rage 27–28; and parents' anxieties 26–27, 28–29; and professional role 26, 28, 32, 33, 34; and psychosomatic approach 31–32, 33; and work groups *see* work discussion groups
Peirce, Charles 144
perception 151–152
perfectionism 93
perinatal depression 36–40, 48; effects of 37–38; and immigrant women 38; risk factors 37; and support networks 37, 38, 43, 45, 46
perinatal period 2–3, 36–50; and co-creation with parents 43–44, 46; early care/intervention project *see* Athens Maternity Hospital project; and multidisciplinary teams 43, 44, 45, 49–50; and premature infants 38, 39, 41, 42–43; psychoanalysts' role in 38–39, 47–48, 49; psychodynamic interventions for 41–48; and relationship models 3, 43, 47
personality disorders 73, 81, 93
personalized medical care 4
phantasies 10, 14, 74
play 63–65
Portmann, Adolf 156
Prato (Italy) 26
pregnant women 3, 36–37, 41–42, 45, 49, 50
premature infants 38–41, 42–43, 48, 53; and mother–infant relationship 39, 40–41; and psychoanalysts' role 38–39
primitive states/defenses 52, 75, 77, 80, 86–87, 134
projection 3, 10, 17, 25, 26–27, 28, 42, 46, 48, 68, 78
psoriasis 142, 146, 147–148, 153–155, 156–157
psychic representations 7, 10
psychic structures 42, 92
psycho-oncology 4, 101–109, 112; and counter-transference 103, 105; and

death anxiety 101, 104–107; and dehumanization of patient 102; and emotions of health workers 102, 103; history/development of 101–104; and living with uncertainty 108, 109; and meaning/value 106–107, 109; movies about 102, 104; oncologists' resistance to 101–102; and positive transference 103, 108; terminal patient case study 107–109
psychoanalysis: neutrality/anonymity in 180, 181, 182; role in medical settings of 1, 38–39, 51–52, 53, 86–87, 162–163; transformative potential of 1, 52, 85, 87
psychoanalysis training 24–25, 102, 103, 166–167
psychodynamic therapy 6, 12, 18, 19, 34, 103, 180; and C-L psychiatry 184; in day hospital treatment 71, 72, 73, 77, 80, 84–85, 86–87; and death/bereavement 112, 114, 116
psychogenic factors 2, 8–12
psychopharmacology 6, 75, 84, 103
psychosomatic approach 2, 6–22, 42, 82, 166, 167–168, 169–170; beginnings of 6–7, 8, 22; and constellative psychomatics 8; and conversion model 8–9; models in *see* psychosomatic models; practical usefulness of 22; and psycho-somatic effects 7, 8–14; and somato-psychic effects *see* somato-psychic dimension; and subjectivity 7, *see also* Balint Groups; Balint, Michael
psychosomatic models 8–14; affect equivalents 9; alexithymia 9–10; and anorexia case study 12–14; of body as locus for enacting relationships 10; as guidelines for MPs 12; practical usefulness of 11–12, 14, 22; and sense of self 11; and therapeutic relationship 12
psychotic symptoms 16, 75, 77, 92, 96
puberty 91, 94
public health 36, 37, 38, 171
punishment, illness as 3

Racamier, P.C. 84
Ramachandran, V.S. 152
Rank, O. 167
Raphael-Leff, J. 42

Rascovsky, Arnaldo 96
Recalcatti, Massimo 92
regression 52, 61, 66, 67–68, 80, 99, 169, 174
relational theory 175, 182
relationship models 3, 43, 47
relationships 10, 14, 87, 98, 115, 116; and skin patients 144, 149–150, 151; symbiotic 21, 144, 153–155
representation 3, 7, 38, 42, 127; and addiction 133–135; alexithymia model of 10; and anorexia 14, 74, 75–76, 77, 78, 79, 80, 81, 82, 85, 87; formal 149–150; object 74, 80; and skin patients 141, 144, 145, 149, 151; in terminal patients 67, 116, 121
Rickman, John 170, 171
Rodriguez de la Sierra, Luis 138
Rogers, Carl 181
Rosenblatt, Bernard 133–134

Sachs, Hans 165
Sampogna, F. 157
Sandler, Joseph 133–134
Saul, L.J. 125
Schacht, L. 168
Schilder, Paul 76
Second World War 164, 165, 173, 174, 183
self: dissolution of 14, 15, 91; sense of 11, 60, 61, 69, 76–77, 82; true/false 133
self psychology 7, 11, 182
self-esteem 13, 67, 76, 79, 81, 106
self-harming 10, 11, 74, 81, 95, 129, 130, 131, 142
self-pity 19, 21
self-representations 3, 10, 67, 82, 156
semiotics 8–11, 144, 151
separation 19, 21, 29, 32, 38, 152, 155
sexual abuse 74, 79, 80–81
Shure, R. 134
Sifneos, P.E. 10, 174
skin patients 141–159; and allergies 5, 142, 143, 148–149; and body boundaries 142, 150, 152; and dermatitis 143, 148, 149, 150, 156; and dermatologists 5, 141, 146, 147–148, 153, 154, 157; and eczema 142, 144, 152; emotions of 143, 149, 150, 151, 154, 155; and environment conception

149; and erogeneicity/eroticism 141, 142, 143–144, 155, 156–157, 159; and Freud 141–142, 143; and the gaze 5, 55–58, 142, 143; and identity 142, 149, 150, 153, 156; interdisciplinary approach to 146, 147–148; and mind/body 141, 142, 143–144; and mirror neurons 151–152; and psoriasis 142, 146, 147–148, 153–155, 156–157; and relationships 144, 149–150, 151; and representations 149–150, 151; and symbiosis/mind–body dissociation 153–155; and symbolization 144, 145–146; and tattoos/self-harm 5, 142, 151, 152; and transindividual/transgenerational transmission 144; and trauma 143
Sloan Kettering Cancer Center (UK) 101, 104
social workers 24, 45, 96, 102, 171, 182
Solomon, Sheldon 106
somatization 3, 10, 144, 177
somato-psychic dimension 1, 7–8, 11, 14–21, 21, 22, 52; and Crohn's Disease *see* Crohn's Disease; and non-compliance 16–18; and skin patients 141, 142, 143–144; and somatic disease as trauma 15–16
somatoform disorders 8, 12
South Africa 52, 62
spirituality 107
Spitz, René 144
splitting 10, 86, 134
Steiner, John 138
Straker, N. 68
subjectivity 4, 7, 22, 50, 92, 119
substance abuse 38, 80, 81
suicide/suicide risk 74, 80, 81, 93–94, 98, 129; assisted 114, 120, 121
symbiotic relationships 21, 144, 153–155
symbolization 9, 74, 81, 82, 92, 117, 134; and skin patients 144, 145–146, 147
Szekely-Kovacs, Alice 164, 165, 170

tattoos 5, 142, 151, 152
Tavistock Institute 24, 25, 165, 170, 171, 173, 174
Tavistock Observation Course 24–25, 27–29
Taylor, G. 7
TFP (transference focused psychotherapy) 83, 87

therapeutic community 72, 75, 84, 85, *see also* Balint Groups
therapeutic relationship 5, 13, 167–168; and addiction 5, 129, 130–132, 135–137; and children with cancer 56–61, 62, 63, 65–66; and eating disorders 94, 98, 99; external/internal elements of 128; and general practice *see* Balint Groups; listening in 1–2; and palliative care 120; and psychosomatic models 12; and Tavistock method 25; and therapist as patient 166–167
Tonnesvang, Jan 126
training 2, 24–25, 45, 72, 96, 102, 161
transference 2, 4, 14, 73, 83, 85, 98, 169, 174, 182; and addiction 128, 135–136, 138; attachment 119; and palliative care 111, 115; positive 103, 108
transference focused psychotherapy (TFP) 83, 87
transgenerational transmission 3, 41, 43, 45, 144
transitional objects 127, 134
transitional space 121, 122
trauma 3, 74, 117–118, 121, 143; and addiction 134, 135; somatic disease as 15–16
trust 12, 18, 132, 134, 136–137, 139

Ulnik, Jorge 152, 156
unconscious 2, 10, 25, 32, 47, 182; and addiction 126, 128, 133, 138; and death anxiety 106, 108, 120; and eating disorder patients 4, 77; and ill children 52, 54, 59, 60–61, 67; and skin patients 142, 144, 147, 148, 158; in therapeutic relationship 128; and transitional space 121
Ungar, Virginia 1
United States (US) 52, 165, 172, 180–182, 185–186

Vienna (Austria) 163, 166
vitiligo 142, 148
Volkan, Kevin 133, 134
von Weizsäcker, Viktor 7

Warburg, Otto 165
White, H.S. 185

whole person medicine 4
Winnicott, Donald 27, 126, 184; and existential maturity 120–121, 126; and infant–mother relationship 127, 168, 171; and object relations 133, 182; and psychosomatic approach 51, 172; and therapeutic relationship 167, 168; and transitional objects/space 121, 127
withdrawal 79, 86

women: and depression 36–37; and eating disorders 80, 91, 95; immigrant 38
work discussion groups 24, 25, 26, 27, 31, 34, 35; and objectivity 33
World War II 164, 165, 173, 174, 183
Wurmser, Leon 130, 132–133

Yalom, Irvin 105, 106
Yeomans, Frank 73